# The
## **Paren**alk
# Guide to
# Your Child and Sex

*Also by Steve Chalke*

How to Succeed as a Parent
How to Succeed as a Working Parent
The Parentalk Guide to the Childhood Years
The Parentalk Guide to Great Days Out
The Parentalk Guide to the Teenage Years
The Parentalk Guide to the Toddler Years
Sex Matters

# The
# Parentalk
# Guide to
# Your Child and Sex

## Steve Chalke

### Illustrated by John Byrne

**Hodder & Stoughton**
LONDON SYDNEY AUCKLAND

First published in Great Britain in 2000
This edition published in 2003

10 9 8 7 6 5 4 3 2 1

British Library Cataloguing in Publication Data
A record for this book is available from the British Library

ISBN 0 340 75661 6

Typeset by Avon Dataset Ltd, Bidford-on-Avon, Warks

Printed and bound in Great Britain by
Bookmarque Ltd, Croydon, Surrey

Hodder and Stoughton
A Division of Hodder Headline Ltd
338 Euston Road
London NW1 3BH
www.madaboutbooks.com

# Contents

## Part Three: The Hot Spots
## – Tackling the Tricky Issues

# Acknowledgements

Thanks to Dave Cody, Maggie Doherty, Richard Gist, Paul Hansford, Tim Mungeam and Jill Rowe for their wisdom, insight and effort in helping to put this book together, and to all the people who offered advice as the manuscript took shape. But most of all thanks to my family – Cornelia, Emily, Daniel, Abigail and Joshua – who every day teach me far more than I could ever teach them.

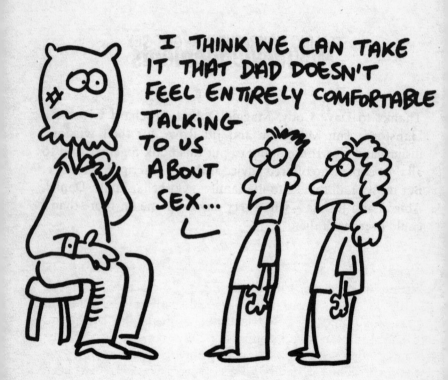

# PART ONE: ENOUGH TO MAKE A GROWN MAN CRY

## TELLING YOUR CHILD ABOUT SEX

# Don't Put It Off, Put It On . . .

## You Can't Insulate Your Child, So Prepare Them

'You're kidding! There's no way my mum and dad would ever do anything like *that*! It's disgusting!'

It was 1965. I was ten years old, standing in a school playground, and my best friend at the time, John Dean, had just told me the awful truth about the 'facts of life'. To be honest, I almost hit him. In fact, the only thing that stopped me was my absolute certainty he was lying. I was sure he'd been watching too much TV and had got it completely wrong. There was no way my conservative, respectable mum and dad would ever be caught dead doing *that*! The idea was just . . . well, unthinkable!

In time, of course, I came to see that John Dean's 'facts of life' theories were right. But, despite obvious evidence to the contrary, as a teenager I was still convinced that my parents were totally ignorant about sex. After all, they *never* mentioned it, and it certainly didn't look as if they ever *did* it. But now I'm a dad myself, and the boot's on the other foot. The responsibility for telling my children about sex is mine, and at last I understand the deep sense of embarrassment that kept my parents' mouths firmly shut on this most intimate of subjects.

The first time I broached the topic of sex with my elder daughter, I was so embarrassed I could hardly speak. In a professional capacity, I'd talked to thousands of young people

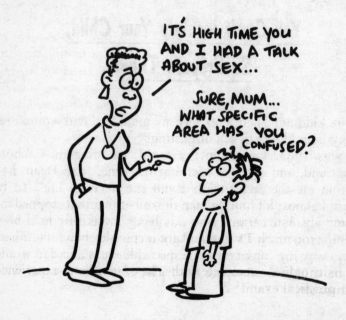

2

about sex without even a hint of embarrassment. I'd even made a sex education video! But this was different. This was my own child. The world suddenly shifted into slow motion, and my tongue felt as dry as a sand-dune in the Sahara desert, hampering all my efforts to get the words out.

The truth is, vast numbers of parents find summoning up the courage to tackle the subject *so* hard to do that they . . . don't! Instead, they opt to cover their embarrassment by avoiding the issue altogether! The good news with this type of approach is, if you adopt it for long enough, you'll eventually succeed in getting yourself off the hook. The bad news is, you'll be opting out of a really crucial part of your child's life. They'll be forced to work out their own beliefs and opinions about one of the most important, sensitive and complicated areas of life with no help, guidance or support at all from you and without the benefit of your wisdom and experience. Don't be fooled: talking to your son or daughter about sex is a tough and embarrassing assignment, but it's an integral part of your job as a mum or dad.

Childhood whizzes by. Before you know it, the kid who wouldn't let go of your leg on their first day of nursery school will have flown the nest, returning once in a while only to eat you out of house and home, clog up your washing machine and recklessly 'borrow' your car whenever you most need to use it yourself. So it's vital to begin the process of talking to them about sex *now*, before the drama of their sexuality turns into a crisis. As hard as it is to do, it's essential for you to take the bull by the horns and start talking to your child about sex before they gain a postgraduate degree in the subject from the 'university of life' – complete with a bit of first-hand experience in the practical exam!

Don't let sex become a 'no-go area' in your child's education – the one part of their life into which you're not prepared to venture, where you fail to give them the kind of help and guidance they vitally need.

 **Top Tip:** *Don't put off talking to your child about sex, and don't make it a 'no-go area' – you'll deprive them of your wisdom and experience.*

### 'We Can Remember It For You Wholesale'

Some parents, of course, are uneasy about actively trying to influence their child's thinking on sex and sexuality. After all, they ask, isn't that just a form of brainwashing?

The simple answer is: *yes*, of course! But then, in a way, so is *every* form of teaching or influence – including school! From teaching your baby daughter basic words to impressing on your forgetful son the vital importance of putting the loo seat up before taking aim and then down again after use, you're constantly attempting to shape and influence the way your child thinks and behaves. That's half of what parenting is about.

What's more, you're not the only one trying to wash your child's brain. In fact, if you're not consciously trying to shape their viewpoint, you're about the only person in their life who isn't. Like it or not, there's a real battle going on to influence what they think. A huge range of people – all with different (and sometimes highly questionable) agendas – are actively competing for your child's mind . . . and money.

So the real question isn't, 'Is my child being brainwashed?' It's, 'What is my child's brain being washed with?' Sexual imagery and influences are everywhere, both blatant and concealed, bombarding your child's brain (and eyes and ears) every single day. No child, from seven or eight years up, can escape our constant talk of sex. It's out in the open and used to sell everything from lager and life insurance to chocolate bars and luxury cars.

- **It's in the adverts.** From hot drinks to holidays, and from prescription-strength drugs to perfume, sex is a vital ingredient in all sorts of advertising campaigns. Ice-cream ads feature perfectly formed semi-naked people eating Maple Nut Crunch in positions that would make a seasoned contortionist wince. Ordinary men become sexual magnets when they acquire the 'Lynx effect', whilst women spice up their fantasy love lives thanks to a can of Diet Coke. The product, of course, needn't have anything to do with sex. In fact, ironically, just about the only things sex isn't used to sell are baby products!
- **It's in the newspapers and magazines.** The Page Three 'stunna' turned *The Sun* into the UK's biggest selling daily paper, making sex a major marketing factor. Now top of the range magazines such as *FHM*, *Vogue*, *Cosmopolitan* and *Esquire* – as well as teen ones like *Mizz*, *Just 17* and *More* – are increasingly explicit in their coverage of sex. No issue is complete without an article on 'Bigger, Better Orgasms' or '15 Sexual Positions for a Monday Morning'. Across the board, the formula is simple: two lines admitting

5

that sex isn't the be-all-and-end-all are swamped by two pages of positions, penises and penetration.

- **It's in the charts.** Since the 1950s, when Elvis 'the Pelvis' Presley's gyrating hips were banned from US TV screens because outraged parents felt they'd prove just too sexually stimulating for their innocent daughters, sex has been an implicit – sometimes explicit – part of rock and pop music. From the subdued sensuality of 'boy bands' setting pre-teen hearts aflutter to the more in-your-face world of pelvic thrusts and groin clutching, sex and romance are as integral a part of pop's image as they are of its lyrics.

- **It's in the bestseller lists.** Sex has always sold literature. From the scandalous poets of ancient Rome to the saucy pilgrims of Chaucer's *Canterbury Tales*, literary 'classics' are often bursting with sexual content and innuendo. Shakespeare's *The Merry Wives of Windsor*, for instance, is the mother of all *Carry On* films, whilst the blatant sexuality of *Lady Chatterley's Lover* outraged 1920s London and led to the book being banned for thirty-five years. Today's writers often rely heavily on sex to spice up their books – even Mills & Boon, famous for their romantic page-turners, no longer stop at the bedroom door.

- **It's on TV and in the movies.** Since the 1970s, few self-respecting films or TV dramas have come without at least *one* eyeball-popping, spectacle-misting, full-frontal sex scene – with all the moans, groans and heavy breathing of a Surround Sound accompaniment. In the soaps, teenagers discuss, not *whether* they should be 'doing it', but when, with whom and how often. And it's almost impossible to walk around your local Blockbuster video store without coming face to face with a dozen tales of sex, secrecy, stockings and suspenders – even if what you were really looking for was Bugs Bunny!

In other words, one way or another, your child is surrounded by images of sex. So trying to influence their thinking isn't the 'interfering' act of a power-mad parent hell-bent on brainwashing their child, but the responsible act of a wise and loving parent keen to help their child develop a balanced perspective on life. *Your* input and influence will help them to make sense of all the other views and opinions that storm them day in, day out.

I once took part in a radio phone-in show based around the issue of parenting teenagers. During the course of the show, one caller attacked me for what he saw as my 'interfering' attitude to adolescents. 'You act like they're not adults,' he remarked, inadvertently hitting the nail on the head. 'That's the whole point,' I replied. 'Adolescents *aren't* adults!'

As the *Oxford English Dictionary* defines it, adolescence is the stage 'between childhood and adulthood'. In other words, teenagers are in-betweeners. Society recognises this by limiting the things they're legally entitled to do, and giving parents and guardians the power and responsibility to make certain decisions on their behalf – decisions they're not yet judged to be mature enough to make for themselves. In other words, though they may *think* they know it all, the truth is that teenagers (just like toddlers) are still learning and they still need your active input and guidance to help them grow from childhood to maturity.

In this, at least, telling your child about sex is no different to telling them about any other part of life. No parent in their right mind would let their teenage son or daughter borrow the car keys so they could teach themselves to drive unsupervised. Apart from being illegal, it's also unbelievably dangerous. In the same way, no parent would calmly let their toddler waltz into the kitchen and play *Can't Cook, Won't Cook* with the carving knives. The harm they could do, to themselves and others, just doesn't bear thinking about!

Let's face it: whether your child is four or fourteen, the fact that you're reading this book at all shows that you already recognise the importance of telling them *something* about sex and sexuality. You don't subscribe to the Free Fall theory of letting them stumble along and experiment with no guidance whatsoever – eventually learning from their own mistakes, but never benefiting from the advantages that come with being able to learn from anyone else's. So don't let your embarrassment stop you from making a vital contribution to your child's development. Without *your* influence, they'll be at the mercy of everyone else's.

---

 **Top Tip:** *If you're not influencing your child's thinking about sex and sexuality, you're about the only person in their life who isn't!*

---

## Faith, Hope and Chastity

Of course, the point of all this 'brainwashing' isn't to make your child's decisions *for* them. It's to help them make their *own* decisions.

Every morning my friend Jason catches the train to his job

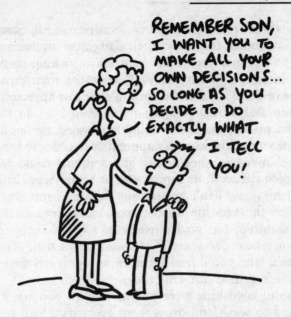

REMEMBER SON, I WANT YOU TO MAKE ALL YOUR OWN DECISIONS... SO LONG AS YOU DECIDE TO DO EXACTLY WHAT I TELL YOU!

in the City, and every evening he comes back to the suburban flat he occupies alone. His routine hardly varies. He never goes out or has friends over for dinner. In fact, he finds it so hard to make friends that he has very few. There's nothing physically wrong with him. He just has no self-confidence or social skills. The reason for this is simple: his doting mother never freed him from her apron strings. She constantly overprotected him, so afraid he might make the *wrong* decision that she never let him make *any* decisions for himself. As a result, when she died, he had no idea how to cope on his own.

In the Middle Ages, many fathers took similar precautions, protecting their children from making the wrong decisions by stopping them from making any decisions at all. Some dads were so concerned to protect their daughters' innocence when it came to sex that they even resorted to locking them up in chastity belts – a guaranteed way to ensure their purity, you would have thought! But the truth is that this approach didn't work then and wouldn't work now. Even back in medieval days, enterprising manacled daughters ended up bedding the handsome young blacksmith's apprentice in order to get a spare key cut. Nowadays they'd just buy a junior hacksaw, learn how to pick the lock, or report you to Social Services!

The truth is, we can't *protect* our children from life, but we can *prepare* them for life. So instead of making sexual decisions for our children, our goal must be to *educate* them to make their own sexual decisions. 'Give someone a fish,' as the old adage goes, 'and you'll feed them for a day. Teach them to fish and you'll feed them for a lifetime.'

When our own kids were young, like all parents, my wife and I used to wash and dress them every day. Sadly, none of them had emerged from the womb with a fully-equipped wash-bag and a working knowledge of personal hygiene, so Cornelia and I had to teach them absolutely everything they needed to know about washing, dressing, using the toilet, cleaning their teeth, combing their hair, tying their shoelaces and generally making themselves look as presentable as possible. Slowly, as they grasped all the essentials (well, most of them), they reached the point we'd been aiming at: DIY, where they could, and would, do everything for themselves.

In the same way, the end-goal of talking to your child about sex isn't for them to obey all your decisions like a mindless robot. Instead, it's for them to make their *own* decisions, and for these to be as constructive, creative and responsible as possible. After all, you don't want them to get hurt, and that's what will happen if they make *bad* decisions. So there's a constant tension between wanting them to make *good* choices and wanting them to make their *own* choices. And the only way to resolve this tension is for you to guide and support them until they're confident and informed enough to make their own decisions *good* decisions – ones they won't regret, either in the morning or five years later.

In a way, it's a bit like equipping them with a kind of internal 'chastity belt' – one for which only they have the key. You want them eventually to replace *your* framework with *their own*. For that, they'll need to know about the range of choices they can make and the possible consequences of each of these choices. But they'll also need the self-confidence to *make* them. So a wise parent does their best to instil in their child the only things that can ultimately help and guide them: wisdom, self-esteem and self-control.

---

 **Top Tip:** *Your task isn't to make your child's decisions **for** them, but to help them make their **own, wise** decisions.*

---

### 'Earth, Swallow Me Up!'

So how *do* you set about providing your child with that much-needed internal 'chastity belt'? A big part of the answer is just to take a deep breath, put your embarrassment behind you and talk to them about sex. Don't worry if the prospect of this makes you feel a bit queasy. No mum or dad ever had an honest conversation with their child about sex and didn't find it a struggle at first just to get the words out, which, of course, is why so many put the whole thing off until it's too late to be of any use, and why others opt for the time-honoured tradition of leaving their child's school and friends to do the job for them.

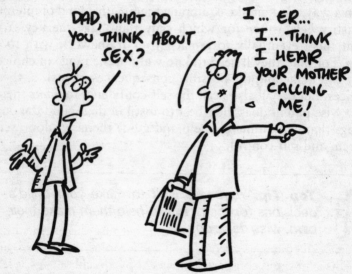

Once relegated to a study of What Goes Where in biology lessons, sex education has now been 'upgraded' to core National Curriculum status. Schools are obliged to teach something of the various emotional and social aspects of sex, not just the basic mechanics. But if you're tempted to think this lets you off the hook, think again. There are at least two good reasons why *you* need to be the first one to tell your child about sex:

1. Poll after poll shows that, with hindsight, *children want their parents to have been the first ones to have told them about sex*, not their school, friends, films, magazines or the media. Mark Twain once defined a 'classic' book as 'something that everybody wants to have read and nobody wants to read'. Sex is the same kind of thing: it's something we all want to *know* about, but none of us actually wants to go through the awkward and embarrassing process of being *told* about it. Even though it's everywhere, sex is still an intensely personal subject – especially during the onset of puberty, when a child's self-confidence is hit hard by the bewildering set of changes happening inside as well as on the outside of their body. Nine times out of ten, your child's desire to know about sex will be hidden behind a thick veil of embarrassment – one that means they'll squirm, frantically avoid eye contact and instantly wish to be somewhere else when you raise the subject with them. But it's vitally important that you do, because the excruciating sense of embarrassment they'll feel learning about sex from you is nothing compared to the embarrassment they'll feel learning about it for the first time in front of their classmates or, worse, finding out that everyone in the class already knows about sex except them!

2. There are bound to be some things *you can explain to your child that they won't learn in school*, especially as you'll be

13

able to give them the kind of one-to-one counselling their school just can't provide. In the privacy of the home, you can raise issues that are just too embarrassing for them to raise in school – from masturbation and menstruation to anatomy or attraction. Few children are brave enough to risk parading their ignorance or misunderstandings in front of friends and classmates by asking too many questions – even if everyone else secretly wants to know the answers as well!

So don't be put off by the wall of silence that might greet you when you raise the subject. Be persistent, and don't be afraid to talk and let your child simply listen, even if they show no outward signs of taking in *any* of what you're saying. Your honesty, and the respect it shows for them, will do a lot.

> **Top Tip:** *Sex is a very intimate, personal subject and your child needs to hear about it from **you** first.*

## 'Education, Education, Education'

But that's not the only reason why they need to talk about sex with you rather than just their friends and teachers. No advice your child is given in the classroom or the school courtyard – about sex, or anything else for that matter – is entirely 'value-free'. A teacher's own moral opinions, for example, will inevitably creep into their lessons, however hard they try to be objective. And since there's no guarantee that you'll agree with an individual teacher's moral values, it's vital for you to present your *own* values alongside those your child will come into contact with at school, in the media, and from their friends. Knowing what *you* think will help them make sense of what other people think, which in turn will help them make up their mind what *they* think. Knowledge, as Francis Bacon once put it, is power.

Your guidance, in other words, will give your child a psychological advantage. It will help prepare them for some of the different views and opinions they'll encounter about sex by equipping them with the kind of moral framework they'll need in order to put everything that's thrown at them into some sort of proper perspective.

Some parents, of course, are so acutely aware of their own past errors that they don't feel confident about giving their child advice about sex. Isn't it rather hypocritical, they ask, to tell their child to 'do what I say, not what I *did*'? The simple answer to this is, *no*. Learning from your mistakes is part of what life is all about. If you can help someone else learn from some of your mistakes as well, so much the better.

So however difficult and embarrassing it is, it's vital for you to learn to discuss the issue of sex within the home, and to start now. The longer you put it off, the more room you give for your child's imagination to run riot, filled with myths and half-truths picked up from elsewhere. I learnt the facts of life in the playground when I was ten, and that was thirty years ago. These days, children as young as seven or eight are being bombarded by sexual images every day, though what they actually pick up at this age is bound to be a mixture of half-truths and total misunderstandings. Even if they're a Junior Einstein, then, your child will *still* get the wrong end of the stick every now and again – like the child who explained to his parents how Sir Francis Drake had 'circumcised the world with a 100-foot clipper'! Without your involvement, there's no guarantee that the misunderstandings won't persist well into their teenage years . . . or beyond!

**Top Tip:** *Knowing what **you** think about sex will help your child make sense of what others think, so let them know.*

## Beat the Rush – Start Early!

The easiest way to beat the cringe factor and start talking to your child about sex is to introduce the subject gently and naturally as they first start asking about where they came from. Don't fall into the trap of saving the whole thing up for a mammoth sixteen-hour 'Big Talk' lecture session – complete with multimedia slide show and hand-drawn diagrams on a blackboard – when they're thirteen or fourteen. Not only will they squirm with embarrassment for the first half hour and then fall asleep for the rest, far more worryingly, they'll probably fail to understand that sex and sexuality are a natural part of life.

So the message is, if your child is still young, start *now*. If they're already a teenager, start *now*. In fact, however late in the day you've left it, the same three golden rules apply.

1. It's better to talk to your child about sex '*little and often*' than all at once. It gives them time to think things through, and slowly builds up their confidence in talking about what can be a painfully embarrassing subject. The more they get used to talking about sex with you, the more they'll feel able to open up and discuss intimate and personal things. What's more, *you'll* get used to talking about it with them. You'll slowly build the kind of trusting relationship that will make talking about sex easier and more effective. In other words, by the time they hit the teenage years it will be a natural subject to chat about.

2. It's important to make what you say *appropriate* to their age and level of understanding. In-depth anatomical descriptions of sex won't make any sense at all to a three-year-old, and will be just as off-putting to a thirteen-year-old if they come out of the blue, in your first conversation with them. Your child doesn't need a crash course in sex. They need an ongoing, on/off conversation. Too much information can be overwhelming and impossible to understand. When six-year-old John asked, 'Where do I come from?', his mum launched into a full and frank biological explanation of egg, ovary, orgasm and intercourse. When she'd finished, half an hour later, John's only comment was, 'That's funny. Peter says he comes from Brighton!' You need to tell your child the truth, but it needn't be the *whole* truth *all at once*. Bit by bit will do fine. Make your explanations simple and straightforward –

17

easy to understand but never the final word.

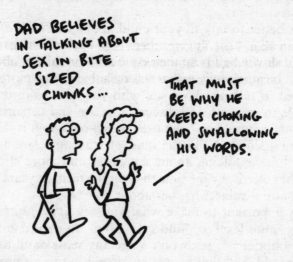

DAD BELIEVES IN TALKING ABOUT SEX IN BITE SIZED CHUNKS...

THAT MUST BE WHY HE KEEPS CHOKING AND SWALLOWING HIS WORDS.

3. If possible, talk about sex *when it naturally arises* in a conversation you're having with your child, or in a question they've asked. As well as saving you from the need to raise the subject out of the blue, it will help them to see sex as a natural part of life. But make sure you avoid making two easy mistakes. First, don't *over*do it, talking about the issue with boring regularity every chance you get, or they'll switch off – when a friend asked his son if he wanted to go for a walk up to the park, the son replied, 'Oh no, dad . . . not *another* sex talk!' Second, don't wait forever for spontaneous opportunities to present themselves – though your aim should always be to talk about sex as it naturally

arises in the conversation, it's far better to 'manufacture' openings than not to talk about it with your child at all!

 **Top Tip:** *Talking about sex isn't easy, so try to build up trust by doing it little and often, in bite-size chunks, rather than all at once.*

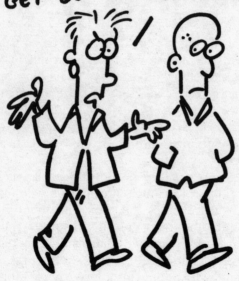

# Knowledge Is Power

## Making Wise Decisions

In his famous novel, *Nineteen Eighty-Four*, George Orwell created a nightmare world in which the government, headed by 'Big Brother', wields absolute power over the people by keeping them in the dark, entirely ignorant of the facts. Not only does Big Brother restrict access to all kinds of basic information, he actively encourages people *not* to find out about the world they live in by assuring them that 'ignorance is strength'.

Tragically, and without meaning to, some parents adopt a similar 'ignorance is strength' approach to telling their child about sex. Keen to preserve the 'age of innocence' as long as possible, and afraid that too much information will push their child into sexual relationships too soon, they choose to put off telling their child about sex until it's absolutely necessary – 'We'll cross that bridge when we come to it,' they tell themselves. It's all done for the best of motives, of course, but the truth is that parents who adopt this approach are more likely to *harm* their child than help them. Far from being a source of 'strength' – or even 'bliss' – ignorance is usually nothing

21

short of a recipe for complete disaster.

For one thing, teenagers can often be remarkably uncommunicative around their parents, especially over something as personal and embarrassing as relationships. They rarely take out full-colour adverts or hire the marching band of the Coldstream Guards to inform you they've just started snogging the most attractive boy or girl in school. In fact, as their mum or dad, you may be the last one to know. So if you're planning to wait until the last minute before 'robbing' them of their precious innocence, you're likely to find that someone else has already put their hands in the till!

What's more, when they *do* start to become preoccupied with sex and relationships, your child's body and emotions will already have begun some radical and confusing changes. All of these changes have to do with their sexuality. So if you've adopted a 'silence is golden' approach, you'll have missed some vital opportunities to help prepare them for the days ahead, and for what it means to begin the slow 'metamorphosis' from boy or girl into man or woman. The more of these valuable opportunities you miss, the harder it'll be for them to feel comfortable about turning to you first – as they *want* to – for the sound advice and support they so desperately crave.

To put your mind completely at rest, the World Health Organisation reports that there's absolutely *no* evidence that sex education leads to more or earlier sexual activity. In fact, all the research actually suggests the opposite – good sex education tends to push *up* the age at which teenagers have sex, not bring it *down*. Being armed with enough information usually delays a child's sexual activity. As the saying goes, 'forewarned is forearmed'!

The truth is, your child's *innocence* is far more likely to be protected if the time bomb of their *ignorance* is removed. Your open and honest guidance will help them make better, more informed, more mature and more responsible choices in the face of enormous pressure from their hormones, their friends and the media.

> **Top Tip:** *Forewarned is forearmed – telling your child about sex is likely to delay their sexual activity, not push them into it.*

## Rights of Passage

When children hit puberty, their hormones suddenly explode. Without warning, millions of these little biochemical messengers run riot in the body, telling individual parts to change from 'child' to 'adult'. Some hormones trigger permanent changes, such as growth spurts. Others regulate how the body works on a day-to-day, week-to-week and month-to-month basis. Oestrogen, for example, controls a woman's reproductive cycle, telling her ovaries to release an egg into the Fallopian tubes every month. Testosterone is the equivalent hormone in men, overseeing sperm production.

Puberty begins for most girls between the ages of about eleven and twelve, though it can be earlier or later. Their breasts start to grow, which is sometimes painful, and they start to develop pubic and underarm hair. It's the understatement of the year to say that all this can make them feel rather awkward and self-conscious. Shortly afterwards – though again, the timing can vary considerably – they begin to menstruate. No matter how well you've tried to prepare your daughter for the onset of periods, this can still be an immensely difficult time. Along with the development of breasts and curvy hips, it marks the end of childhood and the beginning of womanhood.

Boys develop on average a year or so later than girls, at least in terms of visible changes. They begin to grow taller and more muscular, and start growing facial and pubic hair. Their voice drops, as do their testicles, and they enter the highly bewildering world of erections and ejaculations. And, just like girls, their skin often comes under sudden attack

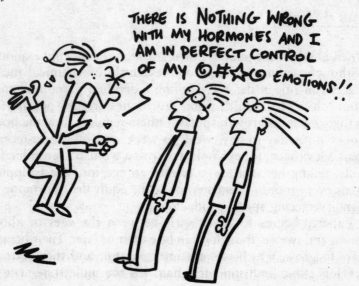

from spots, which erupt like tiny volcanoes all over their face.

But of course, adolescence doesn't stop with Total Body Transformation. These physical changes are dwarfed by the emotional impact puberty can bring in its wake. From hormone-induced anxiety or depression to the general teen battle with self-esteem, adolescence can be a very rough ride indeed. Filled with a range of feelings, urges and impulses they've never experienced before – and usually convinced that no one in the entire history of the world has ever felt them so intensely – they're generally under tremendous psychological pressure.

Having emerged from an age at which any positive physical contact with the opposite sex seemed even less appealing than eating a slug sandwich, they now find themselves coming to terms with distractions and desires that are every bit as bewildering as they are exciting. From *never* having really thought about sex, they suddenly find themselves *always* thinking about sex. From it having being a big turn *off*, it's inexplicably become a big turn *on*.

As their mum or dad, you've got a chance to help them not only *understand* something of these new sensations, but also to be in the driving seat as far as knowing how to *control* them goes. Thousands of years ago, seafarers effectively controlled ships by sheer brute strength. Oars were far more vital than sails, as ancient sailors could only use sails when there was a strong wind blowing in the right direction. If they weren't careful, or took the power of the wind for granted, it could end up taking them miles off course or ripping their sails to shreds. Over time, however, sailors learnt how to control the incredible power of the wind, and harness it so it could be used to drive ships in all but the most extreme conditions. In the same way, it's your role to help your child understand and be able to control their urges and emotions, harnessing the power of their sex drive to work *for* them, not *against* them.

 **Top Tip:** *Your child's hormones will trigger strong urges and emotions – they'll need **your** help if they're to learn how to control them.*

## The Red Badge of Courage

On top of all this, young people live in a society that teaches them they should behave like adults. And to teenagers, the most important part of being an adult is ... sex. Adults appear obsessed with sex. It seems to be the most important thing in the world – why else would it be promoted so much? It seems to be *the* short cut to instant adulthood. It's what adulthood is all about, so until you've 'done it', you're not really mature – you haven't really *arrived*.

Like starting to shave or wearing your first bra, sex is often seen as an official 'badge' of adulthood. Many young people feel that if they haven't yet begun slapping on the shaving foam or strapping on a Wonderbra, they're not as much of a man or woman as those of their friends who have. It can make them feel very left out.

At this age, being average is everything. Not only are girls acutely aware of their own body changes, they're also very keen observers of how these stack up against their friends' progress . . . or lack of it. If you're the first girl to develop breasts, for example, budding or blooming when everyone else is still as flat as a pancake, you're liable to be laughed at; but ironically, if you're the last, still sporting vests or crop tops when your friends are wearing bras, you're equally prone to ridicule. If your bust is bigger – or smaller – than everyone else's, it can make you feel like a freak. The only real insurance against embarrassment and emotional 'exile' is for everyone else to be going through *exactly* the same changes at *exactly* the same pace, constantly maintaining the same standard measurements . . . and that, of course, never happens.

But what's true of 'bits' is equally true of *behaviour*. Having sex can assume mythical proportions. The pressure to do what you think all your friends are doing is intense, even if it turns out later that most of them *aren't* actually doing it! Though research suggests that only one in four boys and one in five girls have sex before the age of sixteen, most fifteen-year-olds are led to believe they're the only virgin left on the face of the earth.

In fact, of course, even if all their friends and peers *were* doing it, it would still make sense for your child to consider all the implications and possible consequences of taking the big step of having sex. By regularly talking to them about it, you can help them balance the emotional pressure they're under from their peers with some common sense and honesty. That way, when they *do* make their decision, it's likely to be one that both their *head* and their *heart* – not to mention one or two other parts of their anatomy – are happy with. After all, they're going to have to *live* with the consequences, so they should at least be aware of them in advance!

***Top Tip:*** *Your child is under big pressure to conform with their friends – it's up to **you** to help them make wise decisions.*

### 'I'll Know What I Think Just as Soon as Someone Tells Me!'

Teenagers, even more than the rest of us, desperately *need* to feel loved and accepted, not least by their friends and peers. It's a vulnerable age. Every teenager is trying to establish who they are as an individual, and what they're worth. Eighty per cent of young people, we're told, are unhappy with their looks: they don't like their nose, their hair, their legs, their colour, their height, their weight, their glasses, their zits or, in some cases, the whole lot! Their self-confidence can be extremely brittle, and their desire for approval can lead them to do things they don't really feel comfortable with, just because they don't know how to walk away with their self-esteem intact.

In the famous old film *Rebel Without a Cause*, James Dean plays a teenage tearaway, confused and confounded by constantly bickering parents. Falling in with the wrong crowd, he ends up getting into real trouble with the police. In a bizarre game of 'chicken', he and another boy drive stolen cars toward the edge of a cliff in order to establish which of them has the courage to stay in the car longest. When the other teenager dies, unable to jump in time, Dean's troubles go from bad to worse. At the heart of it all is a lack of self-esteem. He's so desperate to feel accepted by his peers that he can't walk away from trouble without feeling that he's losing face. As a result, he finds himself doing things he doesn't actually *want* to do, simply because he doesn't know how to say no.

It's exactly the same when it comes to sex. Young people will often do things they don't really *want* to do simply because they need the peer approval that seems to come from doing them. They don't feel strong enough in themselves and their own identity to stand up for what they believe in, regardless of what everyone else thinks. They may know how to form the word 'no' with their lips – after all, they probably say it to you often enough – but they don't always have the self-confidence to say it out loud if it means risking rejection from their friends.

According to the Family Planning Association, about 8,000 girls under the age of sixteen become pregnant in the UK every year. Most of them aren't looking to have sex, much less a baby! By their own admission, they just get carried away, having sex without ever really *deciding* to or even particularly *wanting* to. According to the FPA, the main reason most of them let themselves be swept along in the heat of passion is simple: 'I just didn't know how to say no.' At such a vulnerable time of life, many young people need the reassurance that having sex can offer them – reassurance that they're normal, attractive and desirable. After all, if someone wants to sleep with you, you can't be *that* bad, can you?

So it's not just your child's hormones and peers that can push them into having sex before they'd honestly choose to in an ideal world. It's also their desire to be loved and accepted. Unless they know *you* love them unconditionally, with no strings attached, they may start looking for love in all the wrong places. They may settle for something highly conditional just because being loved by someone – even the *wrong* someone – is better than nothing. So the more you can do to boost your child's self-confidence and self-esteem by helping them see that they really *are* attractive, and that you genuinely love them to bits, the less tempted they'll be to experiment with sex now or in the future as a means of having their personality and looks rubber-stamped and approved by their friends and contemporaries.

> **Top Tip:** The more you can do to boost your child's self-confidence and self-esteem, the less likely they'll be to have sex for the wrong reasons.

## The Right One

As a parent, you walk what can often seem like a tightrope. You don't want to destroy any of the mystique surrounding sex, but you do want your child to see it in its rightful context. You want them to be aware and in control of what they're doing. But it's precisely because you want to retain this mystique for your child that preparing them in advance is so vital.

We all want the first time our child has sex to be special. We want them to be able to look back and think, 'I'm really glad I did that!' Many people's ongoing attitude to sex is coloured by their first time. For some, this will have been planned and prepared for – even long-hoped-for – with the moment, partner, location and atmosphere chosen with care. But for others, the first time won't provide anything like such a pleasant memory. Instead, it will have happened before they felt ready – something they felt they *had* to do because either their partner or their friends pushed them to do it.

So the harder you work at helping your child appreciate their real value and understand the truth about sex and their own sexuality, the more in control they'll be in terms of when, where, why and with whom they first do it, and the more you'll have contributed to their enjoyment not just of the first time, but every time. By talking to them about it on a regular basis, you can help ensure that when they do have sex, it's for the right reasons, with the right person, at the right time, and because both they and their partner genuinely want to.

> **Top Tip:** *By regularly talking to your child about it, you can help ensure that when they have sex, it's for the right reasons, with the right person, at the right time . . . and because they really want to.*

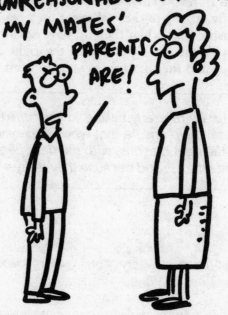

# 'The Good News Is . . .'

## Sex and Sexuality
## Are a Good Thing

'Sex is dirty, degrading and disgusting. So save it for your wife!'

A friend of mine says this was the only bit of advice anyone ever gave him about sex, back in the 1950s. But although he can laugh about it now, he admits that this pathetic explanation left him confused for years. Another friend says that her mother still often tells her, 'I want you to know how proud I am that I was "clean" until I married your father!'

Despite the fact that it's everywhere – or perhaps because of it – sex doesn't have a very good reputation. Maybe it's a hangover from the Victorian era, but we still tend to see it as a bit unsavoury: 'naughty but nice'. For centuries, many of the 'moral guardians' of our society were keen to condemn the whole area of sexuality as a kind of 'necessary evil' – a secret, shameful part of life, even if it was one we couldn't entirely do without. Some Victorians even went so far as to cover over the sexual organs on well-known statues – such as London's famous bronze of Achilles in Hyde Park – that had previously featured naked men or women. Carefully positioned fig leaves were added by people who considered such public displays of nakedness 'indecent', and took it upon themselves to make things 'more presentable'.

Not every country in the world shares our discomfort about sex and nudity, of course. It varies from place to place and culture to culture. Whilst some Middle Eastern countries like to 'cover up' even more than we do, other places around the globe – from the arid plains of Africa to the crowded beaches of the Mediterranean – accommodate partial nudity without so much as batting an eyelid. And the men of some tribes in Papua New Guinea take it to extremes, with a traditional dress code consisting of nothing more than a 'penis gourd' – a hollow tube covering the penis, attached to the body by means of a flimsy leather cord!

It's unlikely to catch on over here, of course. For one thing, the British climate is far too cold – even if the gourd were fur-lined and designed by Giorgio Armani! This is, after all, the land of woolly mittens and wellington boots. For another, it just doesn't fit with the world-famous British 'reserve'. Most of us tend to prefer keeping our assets firmly hidden. But the problem with our rather cloistered approach to nudity and sex, of course, is that it can make us almost ashamed of our sexuality.

Like most parents, Corni and I were perfectly happy for our four children to run around the house and garden in their birthday suits when they were little. What's more, no visitor ever seemed to object to so flagrant a display of naked toddler flesh. It was all perfectly natural. And, whilst we don't encourage them to continue the practice now they're in double figures, we've nevertheless tried to ensure they don't feel ashamed of their bodies or their sexuality. We've tried to place as much emphasis on the *dos* as we have on the *don'ts* when it comes to telling them about sex. Of course we've tried to educate them about the potential problems, perils and pitfalls, but we've also tried to explain that with the right person and in the right circumstances, sex can be not just wholesome but wonderful. We don't want them to grow up with the impression that it's all rather shameful and sordid – not only would they probably fail to get the best out of it, they might even end up feeling guilty about *enjoying* it. And that's more than just unfortunate: it's potentially disastrous.

**Top Tip:** *Be positive – remember that sex is nothing to be ashamed of!*

## A Brief History of Sex

Two centuries ago, before the French Revolution, Pierre Choderlos de Laclos wrote a book called *Dangerous Liaisons* that inflamed and outraged polite society. It tells the story of a teenager, fresh out of convent school, whose sex education has been all about *don'ts* rather than *dos*. Totally unprepared for the passion and strength of her feelings and desires, she can't see how something she was taught was a 'necessary evil' – to be endured for the good of the species, but never enjoyed –

could feel so good. As a result, she's an easy target for a young aristocrat who seduces her, then discards her as soon as he's got what he wants. Times may have changed but human nature hasn't, and thousands of people face exactly the same problems today.

The idea that sex is something we shouldn't ever whole-heartedly enjoy has the weight of many centuries behind it. In part, it stems from the once commonly-held idea that the *real* reason for having sex is to have children. St Augustine – who was every bit the ladies' man before he became a Christian, and once famously prayed, 'Lord, make me chaste . . . but not just yet!' – even suggested it was a sin to have sex for any reason *other than* having children! Thankfully, the rest of the Church and European society through the ages wasn't prepared to go that far – a fact to which, ironically, many of us owe our very existence.

Nevertheless, the suspicion that we shouldn't really enjoy sex has hung around. During the eighteenth and nineteenth centuries, it was common for a husband and wife in polite society to have separate bedrooms. Although people were obviously as interested in sex as ever, few would actually admit to liking it. 'It's necessary in order to continue the human race,' they seemed to be saying, 'but it's messy, and best done at night with the lights off!'

Around 1900, a certain Lady Alice Hillingdon summed up the general attitude when she famously remarked, 'I am happy now that [my husband] Charles calls on my bedchamber less frequently than of old. As it is, I now endure but two calls a week and when I hear his steps outside my door I lie down on my bed, close my eyes, open my legs and think of England.' If the earth moved for Lady Hillingdon, she certainly wasn't letting on about it!

By the 1920s and 1930s, the fashion had changed toward 'twin beds': identical single beds placed alongside one another, often with a bedside table between them. This may have been an improvement, but it still wasn't exactly the height of unfettered passion! At best, young people grew up thinking that sex was society's 'best kept secret'; at worst, they grew up believing that it was something to be *endured* more than *enjoyed*.

With sex now out in the open, you could easily be forgiven for assuming that this way of thinking has been as thoroughly assigned to the vaults of history as Lady Hillingdon herself. But the truth is, it's far from dead and buried. Despite its having found its way into almost every sphere of life, the images associated with sex are frequently negative or manipulative. How often does a steamy sex scene on TV or at the cinema feature a loving husband and wife, for example? Most husband-and-wife bedroom scenes contain books, bifocals and flannelette pyjamas, but rarely even a hint of passion, pleasure or positive sexuality – that's something almost exclusively reserved for torrid affairs.

So whilst sex is beamed straight into your living-room, broadcast across the airwaves and billboarded on to the high street, it's rare for your child to see it reflected positively in the context of a loving, stable relationship. Though most of us would like our children to enjoy a full and happy sexual relationship with one other person for life – let's face it, most of them would like this, too – what they learn about sex from society in general is a long way from this ideal.

In other words, it's not enough to tell your child what they *shouldn't* do when it comes to sex. If you don't also give them a very *positive*, healthy approach to sex and sexuality, you risk leaving them with either very low expectations or a very high guilt factor. If you have a partner, don't be afraid to be a bit lovey-dovey with them in front of your child. Don't be too demonstrative, or they'll just end up reaching for the sick bag. But it's vital to let them see that sex and sexuality are really *good* and that sexual desire won't stop the moment they reach twenty-one or say 'I do'!

---

 **Top Tip:** *If you don't give your child a positive, healthy attitude to sex and sexuality, they'll end up feeling guilty about enjoying it!*

---

## The Whole Story

The truth is, *sexuality* is about more than just sex. It's about being human. Sexuality is part of who we are. It's what makes us male or female. It's everything that goes into making men men and women women, though it mostly finds its expression in the things that make men and women so different from one another: the way we think and feel, and particularly the way we look. Hips, lips, bosom and buttocks are the most obvious physical differences – not to mention genitalia – but in fact almost *any* part of the anatomy can be highly sexual: hands, legs, feet, neck, belly, nose, eyes, ears, hair. People notice and appreciate different things.

What we teach our children about sexuality, therefore, is what we teach them about being human. If we give them the impression there's something inherently wrong with sex, we'll risk leaving them convinced that there's something wrong with them and the way they feel. Sooner or later, your son or daughter will make their own choices about when, where and with whom to have sex. If you want these choices to be informed and responsible, you'll need to talk to them about sex in a positive, natural and guilt-free way. So the first point to get across to them is that sexuality is a *good* thing. It's nothing to be ashamed of, or try to suppress.

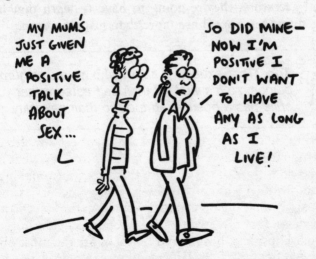

Your child may need to be reassured that if they see an attractive member of the opposite sex across a crowded room and their eyes – or perhaps other parts of their anatomy –

bulge, that isn't 'wrong': it's just good eyesight! Sexual attraction is all part and parcel of being human, even when it's not reciprocated or they're already spoken for.

But, of course, a person's sexuality has as much to do with their character as their carcass. A woman might find a man attractive because he's kind or thoughtful, or makes her laugh, in spite of the fact that he's a dead ringer for the Elephant Man. By contrast, it won't make much difference how beautiful a woman is if she has all the charm, warmth and personality of the Wicked Witch of the West! So if your child is going to find themselves a boyfriend or girlfriend, rather than a mere ornamental accessory, they're going to have to learn that beauty and genuine sex appeal are more than just skin deep.

**Top Tip:** Sexuality is about who we are as human beings, so it's vital for their self-esteem that your child has a positive attitude to their sexuality.

# PART TWO: THE FULL MONTY

## ALL THE FACTS AT YOUR FINGERTIPS

# 'A Funny Thing Happened on the Way to the Form Room . . .'

## The Potential Pitfalls

So if sex and sexuality are such good things, your child may ask, shouldn't they just go out and get on with it? What's to stop them humping and bumping away to their heart's content?

Well, just because something is natural or part of us, that doesn't mean it's always right or healthy to do it. There's a careful line between 'use' and '*ab*use'. Just because we have muscles, for example, doesn't make it right to go around using them to hit people whenever we feel like it. And just because the scientists in *Jurassic Park* had the technology to clone dinosaurs didn't make it a good idea for them actually to go ahead and do it. As one of the characters in the film points

41

out, Jurassic Park's scientists were all so busy finding out what they *could* do, they never stopped to think what they *should* do.

Of course, in *Jurassic Park*, people's mistakes eat them. Fortunately, sexual mistakes are rarely quite so lethal. (Though, as we'll see, sexually transmitted diseases and conditions such as AIDS mean they *can* be that lethal.) Nevertheless, just because sex is basically good, that doesn't automatically mean that every time people have sex it's good. Sometimes the consequences of having sex, even between consenting adults, can be harmful to one or even both of them.

Your child may feel that they're ready for sex. They may definitely *want* to have sex. But however 'right' it feels to them, they still need to think through the possible consequences carefully before leaping into bed with someone. They need to consider where, when, why, how and with whom they have sex, rather than just seizing every opportunity that comes their way indiscriminately.

 **Top Tip:** *Sex is a good thing, but you need to help your child realise that this doesn't mean it's **always** good with **everyone**.*

## A Walk on the Wild Side

We don't have to look very hard to find ways in which sex can sometimes have extremely damaging consequences. There are some very big risks. The first, and most obvious, is the risk of unwanted pregnancy.

Every year in the UK, as we've seen, about 8,000 under-sixteens have their lives turned upside down by becoming pregnant. Some do so deliberately: they want someone to need them or love them unconditionally, and hope a baby will provide just that person. Perhaps they're also looking for a sense of womanhood or independence. Or maybe they just want a baby so much they don't really feel they can afford to wait. The vast majority, however, become pregnant unintentionally. The Family Planning Association (FPA) estimates that of the one in fifteen girls between the ages of fifteen and nineteen who get pregnant, 90 per cent of these pregnancies are accidental.

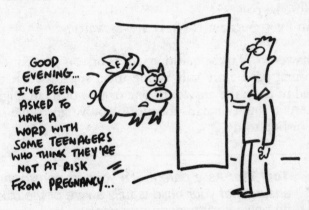

GOOD EVENING... I'VE BEEN ASKED TO HAVE A WORD WITH SOME TEENAGERS WHO THINK THEY'RE NOT AT RISK FROM PREGNANCY...

Most unintentional pregnancies happen because people are uninformed or ill-prepared, so it's vital for you to teach your child the *facts* about contraception and pregnancy. You'd be surprised how many myths, half-truths, old wives' tales and blatant lies are still doing the rounds in teenage circles. The Kinsey Institute – America's famous research institute on sex, gender and reproduction – is inundated every year by letters from teenagers desperate to know the truth about issues to do with sexuality, but too embarrassed to talk to their parents or teachers about it. Amongst the questions they're most constantly asked are:

- Can I get pregnant the first time I have sex?
- Can I get pregnant during my period?
- Can I get pregnant before I start getting my periods?
- Can I get pregnant if I have sex standing up?
- Can I get pregnant if my boyfriend withdraws his penis before he comes?
- Can I get pregnant if I have sex in water?

The answer to all these questions, of course, is yes. But the fact that young people are still asking them suggests that they're tempted to hope the answer to one or two of them might just be no. As a mum or dad, therefore, you've got some serious myth-busting to do.

**Top Tip:** *As a parent, it's your responsibility to ensure that your child is fully aware of the risk of an unwanted teenage pregnancy.*

## Blame It on the Bookie

However, it's not just ignorance of the facts that can lead to an accidental or unwanted pregnancy. An alarming number of teenagers who *do* know about the potential dangers of pregnancy or sexually transmitted disease still take unacceptable risks because, though they know it can happen, they simply don't believe it will happen to *them*.

Few of us are very good at figuring odds. The odds of someone in Britain being struck by lightning, for example, are ten million to one. So it's hardly surprising that few of us bother to protect ourselves against the threat of lightning strikes when we leave home in the morning. We never think it will happen to us, and we're right – it only happens to five or six people a year. By contrast, however, the odds of a girl in the UK between the ages of fifteen and nineteen becoming unintentionally pregnant are a mere seventeen to one. This means that each year about six in every hundred girls of that age get pregnant accidentally!

Some women, of course, can try for years to get pregnant and never succeed. In the end, a number opt for artificial means of insemination such as in-vitro fertilization (IVF), the famous so-called 'test tube baby' method. A smaller number even choose to use a technique called 'artificial insemination by donor' (AID), where their egg or their partner's sperm are fertilized using sperm or an egg donated by an anonymous third party before being inserted into the womb to develop normally. But many other women can get pregnant without even trying and even when they're deliberately trying *not* to.

In just the same kind of way, some men are more fertile than others. Being more fertile doesn't make them 'more of a man', just as being less fertile doesn't make them less of a man. It's simply the way things are. There are many reasons why some people are more or less fertile than others, though few of them are permanent.

My wife, Cornelia, and I have four children, and though *all* of them are wanted, *none* of them was exactly planned. Each came as a bit of a pleasant surprise. In fact, my job meant I had to make so many trips away from home that Corni jokes we only tried it four times . . . with a 100 per cent success rate! But if that's what it can be like for a married couple then in their twenties, who are supposed to know how to use contraceptives, think what it must be like for two teenagers taking their first tentative steps on the sexual superhighway. In truth, less than half of all teenage girls use *any* form of contraception the first time they have sex. As a result, half of all first-time pregnancies occur within about six months of a girl losing her virginity.

 **Top Tip:** *Don't let your child fall for the lie that it could never happen to them – help them to choose with all the facts in front of them.*

## Baby, Baby . . .

There's no more profound consequence of sex than the creation of a human life – whether a pregnancy is planned or accidental.

It's especially true when someone gets pregnant without having given any real thought to what life will be like for the child that ensues. Some very serious thinking needs to take place, as there will be major ramifications whatever course of action a girl decides to take if she finds herself unintentionally pregnant. So whether you've got a son or a daughter, the best time for them to begin the thinking process is *now*, before it's even on the cards.

For those who become pregnant unintentionally, there are basically just three options: termination, giving the child away for adoption, or keeping the child.

**1. Abortion.** There are thousands of abortions every year. More than a third of all pregnant women between the ages of fifteen and nineteen, and half of all pregnant young women between the ages of thirteen and fifteen, end their pregnancy in abortion. In medical terms, this is called a 'termination'. It's a huge decision to have to make. Like all surgery, abortion carries an element of risk and *can* have long-term consequences, including feelings of loss, guilt and remorse, as well as physical side-effects such as internal bleeding or even, occasionally, becoming unable to get pregnant in the future.

Abortion remains a hotly debated issue. Some people are convinced it's morally wrong, whilst others insist that it's a woman's fundamental right to choose whether or not to have a child. But the truth is that most women who have abortions do so because they feel they have *no* choice. It's the only thing they think they can do. Perhaps they or their family just can't afford to bring up a child. Perhaps they're emotionally unready and lack the vital support they know they'll need from their family and friends. There are, to be honest, as many reasons as there are people who have abortions, but almost all of them have one thing in common: if they could see another realistic way out, they'd take it.

You need to explain this fact to your child clearly and carefully, allowing it to impact the choices they make *early on* about whether or not to have sex and in what circumstances to have it, because abortion isn't so much a choice as a sign that your choices have run out.

**2. Adoption.** Most young women decide against a termination of their pregnancy. They feel they want, or have, to see it through to the birth. A number of these, however, choose to give the baby up for adoption after the birth. Some do so because they can't afford to keep the child; some don't want to miss out on their education; some feel they're not yet ready to become a full-time mum; and some believe that others are better prepared and able to give the love and support they feel their child needs.

This is not an easy decision to take, by any stretch of the imagination. It can be totally heart-wrenching to give away a baby you've nurtured for nine months, whether you ideally wanted the child in the first place or not. In fact, some young women find they can't in the end go through with the adoption proceedings and opt to keep the baby anyway. Those who do go through with it can suffer for years afterwards from feelings of grief or remorse.

And it's not just the mums who can be affected by such a far-reaching decision. However loving their adoptive parents might be, most adoptees are filled with questions: why did my mother give me away? Was it my fault? Was there something wrong with me? Some begin a search for their birth parent(s) as soon as they're legally able, at the age of eighteen. (It's illegal for birth parents to make the first contact with their children.) Usually they have one question in mind: why did you give me away? For some children, these are just questions. Others are dogged by feelings of inadequacy, and however irrational these feelings might be, they won't go away.

**3. Adaptation.** Keeping the child, however, isn't an easier option. Pregnancy can be a wonderful experience, but it can equally be painful and uncomfortable. The truth is, it's not only different for different mums, it's different for the *same* mum with different children. Some pregnancies are considerably less problematic and trauma-filled than others.

Morning sickness, backache, food cravings, swollen legs, always having to sleep on your back, always needing the loo (even when you've just been), having to wear unfashionable clothes in unflattering sizes ... pregnant women suffer in varying amounts from any or all of these. With enough emotional and financial support from your family and friends, it can be wonderful. But if there's no one who understands your sudden desperate craving for a charcoal and chocolate pizza, life can be tough. What's more, raising a child is expensive. Even with emotional support, and family members or friends who're prepared to help out on the practical side, being a mum or dad when resources are stretched can be very tricky.

However glad they are that they chose to keep the baby, teenage mothers often mourn the loss of their freedom and social life. It's as though the responsibility of having a baby robs them of being young during the only time in their life when they're actually *allowed* to be young. Their entire world revolves around a tiny person who just eats, sleeps, cries, turns a perfectly ordinary nappy into something that both looks and smells radioactive, and wakes them up in the middle of the night . . . *every* night!

Obviously, *none* of these three options is ideal. But that's why it's so important for you to teach your son or daughter the facts about conception and contraception long before *any* of these options have to come into play. As they say, a stitch in time saves nine!

---

 **Top Tip:** Don't wait until it's too late to teach your child the facts about conception and contraception. Start tackling the subject **now**!

---

## 'It Takes Two, Baby'

Getting pregnant, of course, doesn't just affect young women. So what about the fathers? Though they can't get pregnant themselves, many young men are deeply shaken by the knowledge that they've made someone else pregnant. Some are absolutely delighted, others completely horrified. Some deny reality and act as though it had never happened, or else claim that someone else was really the father. Others face up to their responsibilities.

Thirty years ago, if a boy got a girl pregnant, he was expected to 'do the right thing' and marry her. These were commonly known as 'shotgun' weddings, because it was imagined that if the boy became a little reluctant, the girl's father would march him up the aisle with a shotgun in his back, making him 'an offer he couldn't refuse'! Today, things are much less clear. Boys who impregnate their girlfriends outside the 'bonds of holy matrimony' have no clear influence on what happens next, and their role is very far from defined. Their options, or the options imposed on them, can include, for instance:

- total exclusion
- occasional access to the child
- finding a job to pay for the child's upkeep
- moving in with the girl's parents
- marriage.

It can be a very traumatic and confusing time, and few teenage fathers feel ready to take on the weighty responsibilities of parenthood.

Again, that's why you have to start talking to your son now, before there's a risk of it being too late. Especially toward the lower end of the age range, girls are often reluctant to raise the issue of contraception – which usually means condoms – during a passionate encounter, and guys are often quick to dismiss the suggestion when they do. What's more, they tend to be hesitant about carrying condoms with them, in case they're accused of being a 'tramp'. So talk to them seriously about the need to take full responsibility for their sexual choices, as well as giving them all the information they need on condoms and contraception.

**Top Tip:** *Make sure your child knows that the responsibility for avoiding an unwanted pregnancy doesn't just lie with the female of the species!*

### 'I Left My Heart in San Francisco'

According to the FPA, 54 per cent of all sexually active 16- to 24-year-olds are convinced they're not at risk from getting HIV or AIDS. In part, this is a symptom of the same head-in-the-sand mentality that persuades a similar percentage of them that there's no risk of pregnancy during first-time sex. But if the attitude is the same, the potential outcome of ignoring the risks is considerably more dangerous.

Acquired Immune Deficiency Syndrome, or AIDS, got its name in 1983, when it became clear to scientists not just that it was an identifiable medical condition, but also that it wasn't confined to the homosexual community. Before then, the majority of patients had been gay men in the US, most noticeably San Francisco. Before being called AIDS, the condition was known as Gay Related Immune Deficiency, or GRID. No one knows for sure just how it arose, and there are still big differences of opinion amongst scientists as to exactly what it does and how to fight it. But one thing is clear: it's no longer a 'gay plague', if it ever was. The majority of AIDS sufferers are now heterosexuals living in central Africa.

When a person has AIDS, their immune system – the body's way of fighting disease – stops functioning properly. It's a condition, not a disease. Nobody actually dies from AIDS itself; instead they die from secondary diseases, like pneumonia, which are usually curable in people whose immune systems are firing on all thrusters. At its root is a virus – HIV, the Human Immunodeficiency Virus – that attacks a person's immune system, causing them to become unable to fight off disease.

Although deadly, HIV is a 'brittle' virus, which means that, unlike many other viruses, it can't survive long outside the body. Because of this, there's no danger of it going airborne or spreading either infectiously (through proximity) or contagiously (through touch). It can only be passed from one person to another by means of exchanging actual bodily fluids like sperm or blood. And since blood for transfusions is now routinely screened to detect the presence of HIV, the main ways a person can get AIDS are through sharing equipment used in injecting drugs like heroin, or through having sex with an infected person.

Because HIV doesn't turn people lime green or make them grow an extra head, it can be very difficult to know who has it. Like most viruses, it can have a long incubation period, which means it's possible for people to carry HIV in their body for years before developing AIDS. In fact, scientists now suspect that some people will be 'carriers' of the virus without *ever* developing AIDS. This means, of course, that you can have HIV without even being aware of it. What's more, HIV doesn't discriminate. It will attack anyone. It doesn't matter if you're young or old, male or female, black or white, homosexual or heterosexual. It makes no difference if you've lived a life so bad it would have made Hitler blush or so good it would have sent Mother Teresa green with envy. And it makes no difference at all whether you've had sex every day, twice a day, for umpteen years or are having it for the first time. The chances are exactly the same. If you have sex with someone who is carrying HIV, then you risk getting it yourself. And that can eventually lead to AIDS.

> **Top Tip:** Make sure your child knows the facts about AIDS – don't let them die of ignorance.

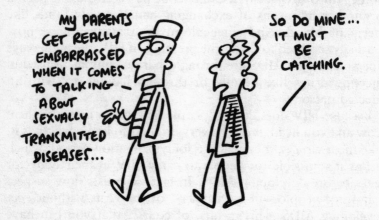

## The Not-So-Magnificent Seven

In recent years, AIDS has tended to hog the headlines as far as sexually transmitted diseases (STDs) go. Yet it's very far from the only disease your child risks getting if they indulge in unprotected sex. In fact, it's estimated that each year UK hospitals treat about 500,000 new cases of other STDs. Of the seven most common, two, like AIDS, are caused by viruses for which there is still as yet no cure, whilst the other five are the result of bacterial infections, usually treated with penicillin or other antibiotics.

- **Herpes** (viral) causes the skin around the genitals to itch and burn. Clear blisters appear, sometimes along with headaches, fever and muscle aches. Symptoms tend to disappear within three weeks, but the virus remains dormant in the body, and can recur at any time.
- **Genital Warts** (viral) are soft, painless warts growing on or near the genitals. More of a nuisance than a problem, they can nevertheless be a factor in the later development of cancer of the cervix or the penis. Though they can be removed in the same way as other types of wart, there is no cure for the virus that causes them.
- **Syphilis** (bacterial) presents early symptoms of hard, painless ulcers around the genital region. If untreated, this can develop into the presence of a fever, headaches, sore throat and skin rashes. Symptoms then seem to go away, but in one third of cases come back, sometimes doing serious damage to the heart or the nervous system.
- **Chancroid** (bacterial) is an ulcer either on the penis or near the vagina, which fills with pus and is very painful.
- **Gonorrhea** (bacterial), commonly known as the 'clap', begins with a burning sensation when passing urine, and the production of a yellowish liquid seeping from the opening of the urethra (the tube taking urine from the

bladder to outside the body). If untreated, it can sometimes spread back up the body to cause inflammation of the prostate gland in men or Pelvic Inflammatory Disease in women.

- **Genital Chlamydia** (bacterial) has symptoms very similar in most cases to gonorrhea.

- **Pelvic Inflammatory Disease** (bacterial), most often caused by gonorrhea or chlamydia, involves the Fallopian tubes becoming infected and even scarred. It can cause an abscess (pus-filled swelling) in the ovaries or Fallopian tubes, and pain during sex. It increases the risk of infertility and ectopic pregnancy (where the foetus grows outside the womb).

In addition to this, the risk of developing cervical cancer is now reckoned to be doubled in women who begin having sexual intercourse before the age of seventeen. It's also thought to be increased by having sex with a number of different partners.

It's not vital for your child to know the ins and outs of every sexually transmitted disease off by heart, so there's no need to replace their traditional bedtime book with an up-to-date copy of *Dorland's Medical Dictionary*. Your aim is to *inform* them, not frighten them into becoming a monk or a nun! They need a proper grasp of the potential pitfalls of making the *wrong* choice when it comes to deciding when, where, how and with whom to have sex. That way, there's a good chance of them making the *right* choice!

**Top Tip:** *Your aim is to inform your child, not frighten them. Give them enough facts to make a wise and informed decision.*

### 'One Small Step for a Man, a Giant Leap for Mankind'

But, of course, not all the harmful effects of sex with the wrong person or at the wrong time are physical. For lots of people, its emotional effects can prove just as hurtful.

When a person is 'in love', sex can seem like the natural thing to do, the logical 'next step' in a relationship. But it's a big step to take, often heightening and complicating their emotional involvement with their boyfriend or girlfriend. If this is just one-sided, or the relationship is short-lived, it can leave them feeling hurt or betrayed, their self-esteem hitting rock bottom.

For lots of young people, their first experience of sex isn't planned. They just get carried away, or their boyfriend or (occasionally) girlfriend pushes them into it as 'proof' of their love. As a result, they can end up with mixed feelings about the whole thing because they weren't ready for it. Their first experience of sex ends up being damaging because it took place in the wrong way, at the wrong time and often with the wrong person. It was meant to be a special experience, but actually it turned into something harmful and negative.

Sex isn't a sport like football. It's not a sign of physical maturity like shaving or growing breasts. And it's not a proof of love like a ring or a Valentine's card. It's about sharing who you are with another person on a very intimate level, and it should be chosen freely by both parties. Tragically, this isn't always the case. As well as people feeling pushed into having sex, an alarming number are forced into having sex against their will.

So whilst we all have sexual desires and drives, clearly not every expression of them is good. Sex may be natural and healthy, but we still have to treat it with care – just as we'd treat anything else of value. We can't behave recklessly without suffering the consequences. We're not just flesh and bone. We're people with emotions and feelings.

Your child needs to see that sex, as an intimate act between two people, can't simply be reduced to a physical activity. We instinctively know that it means more than that. They also need to realise that their sexual decisions aren't just personal. They can have important implications for others, for their families and for the whole of society. A few minutes of fun can result in the creation of a human being with a lifespan of eighty years or more, who may in turn have children of their own. Long after they're gone, in other words, your child's actions could still be having repercussions . . . good or bad. So it's very important for them to think about how their decisions will affect others *before* they make them.

 **Top Tip:** *Sexual decisions have consequences – as a parent it's your task to help your child think through the implications of their decisions.*

# Here's One I Made Earlier

## An A to Z of Contraception

Picture the scene . . .

It's Friday night, you're out for the evening, leaving your child home alone with their boyfriend or girlfriend. They've shoved some smoochy music on the CD player and they're soon in each others' arms . . . and throats . . . and . . .

Now if we're honest, when we have the hots for someone, we know there comes a point when our brains shut down and we find it very difficult to control our desires. No matter how self-disciplined we are, we can easily forget it all when our hormones take over. Of course, we never *mean* it to happen this way. Things just go too far. In fact, according to the FPA, almost a third of all pregnant teenagers get pregnant simply because they 'get carried away' and don't know how to stop.

The truth is, there are two very simple ways to avoid unwanted pregnancies (as well as some of the other less desirable consequences sex can have): use contraceptives or don't have sex.

Some parents are understandably worried that encouraging their child to use contraception is basically the same as encouraging them to have sex. Won't *having* condoms, they ask, push them into *using* them? For some it's a moral issue, whilst others are simply concerned not to influence their child to have sex with the wrong person, or before they're good and ready. But that's exactly why it's important to tell your child about contraception in such a way as to encourage them to think carefully about the possible consequences of having sex *before* they decide whether or not to do it. After all, your basic aim in telling them about contraception isn't to give the green light to their sleeping around just so long as they use a condom. It's to reduce the risk of them rushing into an unthought-through relationship, and to help them take a more responsible, longer term view.

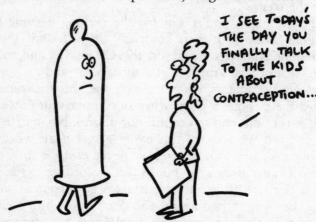

I SEE TODAY'S THE DAY YOU FINALLY TALK TO THE KIDS ABOUT CONTRACEPTION...

A wise parent therefore adopts a kind of belt-and-braces approach, presenting the facts about the various different types of contraception available – and why they could be a real lifesaver – alongside moral, social and emotional arguments as to where, when, how, why and with whom sex can best be enjoyed. This way, your child will begin to understand how contraception fits into the overall picture of their sexuality before making their own informed – and hopefully *wise* – decisions. In addition, a wise parent helps their child to develop the self-confidence needed not just to make their decision, but to stick to it once it's made. So, as vital as it is, information about contraceptives needs to form just one level of an intentionally multi-layered approach.

---

 **Top Tip:** *Be careful to avoid the two extremes: telling your child nothing about contraception and telling them about nothing **but** contraception.*

---

### Keep Taking the Medicine

There are ten commonly recognised forms of contraception. Each has its own unique set of advantages and disadvantages, though it has to be said that some are far more effective than others. So counting down in order of effectiveness, here are the 'top ten'.

**10. The Quick Retreat.** Withdrawing the penis during sex, before ejaculation, is known by the Latin term *coitus interruptus* (literally, 'interrupted sex'). It's said that during the Middle Ages, when adultery was universally understood to be a terrible sin, wealthy men would order their servants to interrupt them as they were having it away with their mistress, as they believed that if they didn't ejaculate, it wouldn't count! However, *this has no value at all as a contraceptive method . . .* as their umpteen illegitimate children proved. Although the sperm ejaculated during sex won't enter the womb if the man withdraws before the end, the failure rate is still between 20 and 25 per cent. This isn't just because the timing is hard to get right. It's also because the tiny amounts of sperm-filled lubricant emitted by the penis *before* a man reaches his orgasm can be enough to make a woman pregnant.

9. **The Sponge.** This soft sponge, filled with spermicide, acts like a less-efficient version of a diaphragm, with a failure rate of between 10 and 25 per cent. Like the diaphragm, it cuts down on the spontaneity of the occasion as it has to be inserted into the vagina just prior to sex.

8. **The Diaphragm.** This rubber cap, shaped like an old First World War army helmet, is placed inside the vagina, over the cervix, and used with spermicide. It has an estimated failure rate of between 4 and 18 per cent.

7. **The 'Natural Method'.** Counting the days, as well as recording body temperature and other signs that a woman is at her most fertile, and avoiding sex at this time has the unique distinction of being the only method of contraception endorsed and approved by the Roman Catholic Church. Nevertheless, it still fails between 2 and 20 per cent of the time.

6. **The Condom.** This is a thin sheath of rubber that lines either the penis (male condom) or vagina (female condom) like a thin, transparent rubber glove, collecting sperm before it has a chance to enter the womb. This is the only form of contraception that can protect against HIV infection. Condoms come in a range of colours, sizes (small condoms are often sold as 'snug-

fitting' or 'contoured'), thicknesses and, for use in oral sex, even flavours! But whilst they're about 98 per cent effective when used by adults, the FPA estimates that when used by teenagers the failure rate can be as high as 15 per cent.

**5. The Pill.** There are actually two *basic* types of contraceptive pill, and several different *sub*types. Scare stories about links with cancer haven't been substantiated, but whilst the pill is estimated to have a failure rate of less than 1 per cent if used carefully, a woman does have to remember to take it regularly. Missing just one day jeopardises the entire month's protection.

**4. The Injection.** A semi-permanent contraceptive for women, this is a slow-release hormone, good for two or three months – but not for the squeamish! Its failure rate is about 1 per cent.

**3. The Implant.** Similar to the injection, this is a slow-release hormonal implant for women, slipped under the skin of the upper arm by a doctor and good for five years, again with a success rate of around 99 per cent.

**2. The Intra-Uterine Device.** The IUD, a T-shaped plastic and copper gadget inserted into the womb for five years, works by stopping a fertilised egg from being able to implant itself and grow on the lining of the womb. It occasionally causes scarring of the Fallopian tubes, but has a normal failure rate of around 1 per cent.

**1. The Final Frontier.** As this method involves surgery, it's not for the faint-hearted or indecisive, and definitely not for teenagers! In women, the Fallopian tubes connecting the ovaries to the womb are cut or blocked. It's called 'female sterilisation' or 'tubal ligation'. In men, the *vas deferens* connecting the testes to the penis are snipped. This is known as a 'vasectomy'. These operations are permanent, although a reversible form of the operation is available for women. The failure rate is approximately 0.1 per cent.

In addition to these, there's the so-called 'emergency pill', which can be used up to three days after sexual intercourse to prevent the fertilised egg from attaching itself to the wall of the womb. It's roughly 96 per cent effective, but doctors are concerned that some women are using it as an alternative to regular contraception. They're far from convinced that this is safe, as it was designed only for *emergency* use, and hasn't yet undergone the rigorous testing needed for *regular* use.

Contraceptives, of course, are designed to stop a woman from getting pregnant. Except for condoms, which were designed specifically to stop the spread of STDs, none of them give any protection whatsoever against HIV and AIDS. And none, including condoms, are 100 per cent effective. Contraception may help to make sex 'safer', but, as the World Health Organisation makes clear, it can never make it totally 'safe'. In fact, the only tried and tested, positively guaranteed method of preventing pregnancy is: don't have sex!

---

 **Top Tip:** Contraceptives vary considerably in style and effectiveness, and abstinence is the only fully guaranteed method.

---

## Safe Sex?

As far as AIDS is concerned, of course, there's no cure, so prevention is everything. Just as there are two ways to avoid getting

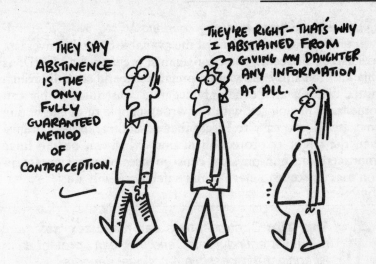

pregnant, there are two ways to prevent yourself from becoming 'HIV positive': always use a condom or never have sex with anyone who might possibly have the virus. But, of course, it's hard to know who has been sleeping with whom. People often lie about their past misadventures, so it's difficult to know who has the virus, especially since it can take years to show itself.

The evidence so far is that the failure rate for condoms in preventing the spread of AIDS is the same as their failure rate in preventing pregnancy. So the only sure-fire way of not getting AIDS is only ever to have sex with someone who only ever has sex with you (and *has* only ever had sex with you). As the World Health Organisation suggests, '*The most effective way to prevent HIV transmission is to abstain from sexual intercourse, or for two uninfected partners to remain faithful to one another. Otherwise the risk of spreading HIV can be*

65

*significantly reduced by using condoms.*'

But recognising that none of the available contraceptives can give us 100 per cent protection against pregnancy and AIDS is only half the story. Unwanted pregnancies and sexually trans-mitted diseases aren't the only negative consequences that can come from having sex with the wrong people or at the wrong time. It's all too easy to forget that no contraceptive can give even the slightest protection against what can be the huge emotional and non-physical consequences of sex. Contraception may make sex safer . . . but safe? Definitely not!

---

 **Top Tip:** *Contraceptives can make sex 'safer', but never entirely 'safe', and they can't protect at all against the possible emotional dangers.*

---

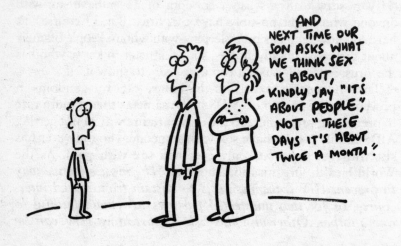

AND NEXT TIME OUR SON ASKS WHAT WE THINK SEX IS ABOUT, KINDLY SAY "IT'S ABOUT PEOPLE", NOT "THESE DAYS IT'S ABOUT TWICE A MONTH"!

# What's Love Got to Do With It?

## The Emotional and Relationship

## Sides of Sex

James Bond entered the room, silently pulling his trusted Walther PPK from its holster. He was tall and exceptionally handsome, with a cruel but tender smile. The beautiful girl, dressed in the same evening-gown she'd been wearing when he'd caught sight of her earlier, was draped seductively across the bed's luxurious silk sheets. She looked up at him demurely and fluttered her long, dark eyelashes. Closing the door, he put the gun down on the table.

'Hello,' she whispered, in a voice that could melt butter. Bond crossed to her and smiled, cruelly but tenderly.

'The name's Bond,' he said, confidently. 'James Bond.' He kissed her passionately.

'Take me,' she breathed, effortlessly slipping out of her clothes. 'Oh James, be cruel but tender with me . . .'

We all know how fake the world of James Bond is. In Bond's world, sex is always wonderful and it comes with absolutely no long-term consequences. No one seems to have heard of condoms or AIDS. The women who fall into his arms never have periods, or headaches, or moods, and change with every film. He's always muscular and his women are always beautiful. No one's ever tired or tense. Bond never gets cramp in full flow, or fails to perform, and the women always have fully vocal, earth-moving multiple orgasms. What does it matter, you might ask? After all, this is the movies, this is fantasy land . . .

Well, as strange as it may seem, the problem is that many of us actually end up half-believing that it's true. We seem to *expect* that, at least where sex is concerned, real life should be like the movies, and suspect that this is exactly the way it is for everyone except us. But the truth is that Bond's bedroom scenes, like virtually all movie sex scenes, sell you a soft-focused, fully orchestrated, Surround Sound . . . lie.

Of course, sex is often a wonderful experience. But it can equally be . . . well . . . messy. The sheets are cold, people often aren't in the mood, hair gets in the way, the phone goes at the wrong moment, one of you is tired or has eaten too much, and someone has to sleep in the damp patch. It can be very tender and romantic, but it can also be ordinary, mundane, humiliating, ungratifying, unfulfilling, uncomfortable, disappointing . . . even boring!

Fuelled by the outlandish boasts of their classmates, your teenager may well imagine that having sex round the back of the bike sheds will cause the earth to move, heavenly choirs to sing, angels to weep and wise men from the east to turn up with gold, frankincense, myrrh and the obligatory post-coital cigarette. But, in reality, the only things that are likely to move are the bikes as they crash down on top of them!

So, as a parent, it's your job to put right some of the wrong impressions about sex that your child, like any other, is bound to have picked up. You'll have to explain that:

- like so much in life, getting the most out of making love takes practice, patience and persistence
- sometimes one partner – and it's not always the man – is more in the mood than the other, who may need to be slowly and sensuously warmed up to the idea
- men and women often enjoy different things about sex, bringing different expectations with them
- whilst men nearly always achieve orgasm, the same can't be said for women, which can leave both of them feeling like they've somehow failed
- the simultaneous orgasm, a vital part of any movie sex scene, is very much the exception rather than the rule.

 **Top Tip:** *Telling your child about sex involves telling them about the squishy, squelchy moments as well as the tender, romantic ones.*

## Things That Go Bump in the Night

Sex is more than just a biological act and we're more than biological machines or robots. Sex involves not just *motions* but *emotions*. As humans, we're more than a collection of minerals and bodily fluids. We've got a soul – the thing that makes us who we are, with all our particular characteristics, our likes and dislikes, our feelings and emotions. And this means that sex is always more than bonking. It's an act that unites two people. It's a moment when 'two become one'.

To be enjoyed at its best, as most of us realise, sex needs to take place within the context of a long-term, committed and permanent loving relationship. Most children understand this fairly well, though they may have difficulties with the concept of 'long-term'. They are, after all, the same child who plaintively used to ask, just two minutes into an arduous two-hour car journey, 'Are we *there* yet?' When they hit the teenage years, and their hormones hit them, you may find that their idea of a long-term committed relationship rapidly shrinks from a whole lifetime to anything in excess of three weeks! They'll need your help to see their relationship in its long-term context before making any big decisions.

This means it's no good waiting until the tornado hits and *then* trying to get the message across. They'll probably be so swept away by the force of their emotions that they won't be able to hear your words of wisdom. What's more, rather than seeing your 'topical' advice as being about relationships in general, they may take it as a personal attack on their *present* relationship, or a sign that you don't trust them to make their own decisions. So, long before they get into this situation, they need to have understood from you that what looks good in the immediate future may not always turn out to be so fruitful given the fullness of time – all that glitters isn't gold.

To get the best out of sex, for example, two people need to love and trust each other enough not to worry or blame each other when it goes wrong, as it inevitably will from time to time. It should never be a way of satisfying their own desires. Sex is about giving as well as receiving. It needs two people who are willing to learn about each other, taking the effort to find out what brings them pleasure.

But it's not just practice and patience that make sex most satisfying. It needs to be with someone you love, trust and respect. It's about sharing yourself intimately with another person. And as this kind of sharing makes you vulnerable, you need to be sure they won't take the opportunity to hurt you. That's why the shallower the relationship is between two partners, the shallower the sex will be, however good it may feel at the time. And by the same token, the deeper the relationship is, the more meaningful the sex will be.

This kind of trust, of course, takes time . . . and commitment. When asked who he thought Hollywood's greatest lover was, one star replied that it wasn't promiscuity or sexual technique that made a lover great – it was their ability to love one person well for forty odd years. 'Anyone can sleep around,' he added. 'Even dogs do that!' That's why, throughout history, most people and cultures have found that the best context for sex is a long-term, committed, loving relationship.

However you slice it and dice it, in the end we're basically talking about the idea of marriage.

 **Top Tip:** *Your child needs to understand that sex is more than bonking – it's about love, trust, care and commitment.*

## Horse and Carriage

Throughout history, the world has always had, as part of its system, the idea of committed, permanent relationships. It's not a modern thing, nor is it a particularly European or even a Christian thing. The ancient Greeks had marriages, as did the Egyptians, the Romans, the Syrians, the Assyrians, the Babylonians, the Barbarians, the Byzantines, the Persians, the Picts, the Angles, the Saxons, the Anglo-Saxons, the Huns, the Goths, the Visigoths, the Ostrogoths . . . you get the idea. Even now, every society, culture and country on earth has its own codes about relationships, and they *all* include the idea of marriage – a permanent, committed and loving relationship between two people.

What's more, most cultures, whatever their religious background, have historically had laws forbidding hanky-panky outside marriage. In some, the punishment for adultery was very harsh indeed – sometimes even the death penalty! That's a very big price tag for a few moments of stolen pleasure, and it certainly seems steep today, given the ease with which people jump in and out of bed with each other, married or not. But however tough or unjust these punishments now seem, their aim was simple: to keep sex within marriage.

Why should this be? After all, marriage has a pretty bad press. More than a third of all marriages in the UK end in divorce, and many of those that remain intact still fail to rate highly on the 'eternal bliss' stakes. Somewhere along the line, love and romance seem to turn into habit and toleration. For every marriage we know that has worked, most of us can think of one or two that haven't.

72

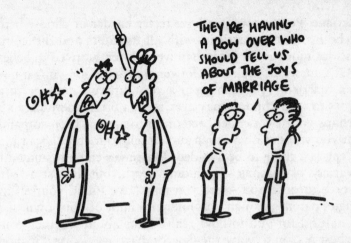

But if marriage is really so *bad*, why do we see it cropping up so consistently throughout history? Surely someone, at some point, could have called a halt and said, 'This is stupid! Let's sit down and come up with something better!' For example, what's wrong with a kind of non-renewable, fixed-term three-year contract, with shared living quarters, equal choice of television programmes, agreed division of the household chores, comprehensive bedroom rights, and a built-in opt-out clause for either side after eighteen months? Why hasn't something like this caught on? Why do people still make permanent vows, even though there's a one-in-three chance of the marriage ending in court rather than at the crematorium? And why do some couples who *haven't* gone through the marriage ceremony nevertheless live together long-term exactly as if they *had*?

Perhaps the truth is that there *is* no better system than

marriage. Perhaps we just have to try harder or choose better. Or both. Maybe marriage, with all its faults and difficulties, has a lot more going for it than we've often been led to believe.

Of course, if you're no longer married – or you've never been married – this can seem a very difficult message to get across to your child. It may even seem a bit hypocritical to try. Perhaps your own experience of marriage has been so painful that you wonder if you even *should* tell your child about it . . . except as a thing to be avoided. Marriages come to an end for a variety of reasons – including death, but almost as often divorce or desertion – and you may have found yourself as a 'single' parent through absolutely no fault of your own. If so, it's natural for you to have real doubts about whether you're the best person to wave the flag for marriage . . . or if it should be waved at all.

But the truth is that, whatever your marital status – whether you have or had the best marriage in the world, or your marriage broke up, or you've never been married – you're *still* the best person to tell your child about the way it *can* work and the security it *can* provide. After all, you're the one person they know who loves them unconditionally. And despite its high failure rate, at heart marriage is about loving and being loved unconditionally and exclusively by one person for life. And that's something most of us want for our children . . . and ourselves.

 **Top Tip:** *Whether you're married or not, it's wise to teach your child what so many different cultures have seen in it for so long.*

## Four Play

'Marriage,' some people argue, 'is only a piece of paper.' Are they right? Well . . . no. The truth is that the piece of paper – the marriage certificate – is actually no more than a symbol of everything else that marriage is about. Neither is marriage about a simple ceremony, a white dress, relatives you haven't seen in twenty years, cake, endless photographs, awful hats, boring speeches and twenty-six toasters. *That's* a wedding!

Marriage is about a lot of things, but four come particularly to mind: friendship, support, family life and commitment.

**1. Friendship.** Above all, husbands and wives are friends and companions. They love one another, which is, perhaps, the highest form of friendship. A husband or wife should be your best friend – someone with whom you can discuss all your problems and share both the good times and the bad times. They should be someone who grows to the point where they know you intimately and love you for exactly who you are without reserve.

**2. Support.** A friend also supports you. You know you don't have to be on top form all the time because, when things go wrong and times are rough, friends are there to pick you up – or at least be there for you. When you marry someone, you vow to love and support them *forever*, come what may. A wife or husband is a partner who's committed themselves to giving you the support you need for as long as you're both alive.

**3. Family life.** Marriage creates the best environment for family life. Of course, single parents have proved very effectively that families don't have to be 'nuclear': mum, dad and two point four kids. In fact, many lone parents bring up their children with more love and security than other more 'traditional' families. But even most single mums and dads agree that the *ideal* situation is a stable environment with both mother and father present. It may not always work out that way, of course, but it's the gold standard to aim at.

**4. Commitment.** Perhaps the most important thing about marriage, though, is the public commitment each partner makes to love the other regardless of what the future holds. In a wedding service, the bride and groom promise to remain together 'till death us do part'. In our disposable society – in which, if you get fed up with something, you trade it in for a new one – there's a real temptation for us to treat people like objects, part-exchanging them for a different model whenever they don't match our expectations, turning *Mr* or *Ms Right* into *Mr* or *Ms Right For Now* . . . until someone better comes along. By contrast, marriage – with its promise to remain true to the other person no matter what – helps us treat them like human beings.

A Nobel Peace Prize winner was once interviewed for television. In his eighties, he'd been married for over fifty years. When the interviewer asked if he thought his wife was the most beautiful woman in the world, he replied, 'Of course not. She's eighty! But she *is* the woman I love the most, the one I'm committed to.' Marriage is about putting your money where your mouth is. It's about making a *public, permanent* commitment. And in our ever-changing world, it's the quality and content of our commitments that define who we are.

**Top Tip:** *Marriage isn't a piece of paper – it's a permanent, passionate friendship. That's why it's the best context for sex.*

## More Than Meets the Eye

We're all looking for love. That's why it's such a tragedy when we settle for nothing more than sex or romance, however enjoyable these things may be at the time. Eventually, we're just left feeling empty, cheated and bitter. There's a lot more to love than going to bed with someone. The fact is, for any relationship to work it has to be based on security and trust, built on the foundation of a mutual commitment to remain faithful to one another.

That's why sex is at its best and most fulfilling within marriage. Sex is about more than itself. It's both a physical and an emotional experience. It's about the *people* who have sex, and the way they feel about each other, rather than the physical act itself. It's not primarily about humping and bumping, as if memorising the *Kama Sutra* and training for Olympic Gold in gymnastics was the way to achieve a fulfilling sex life. At heart, it's about love and security. In the end, what really makes sex fulfilling isn't technique or fitness. It's not size or strength. It's not even beauty. It's the people who have sex, and the relationship they have with one another. It's sharing who you are totally and intimately with another person.

So the ever-popular question, which your child may ask –

77

'Don't we need to find out if we're sexually compatible before we get married?' – misses the point. If you're compatible in other ways, you'll be compatible sexually. And if you're not compatible in other ways, no matter how good the sex may be at a technical level, it will never be enough. Sex is at its best when it's with someone you love, trust, support and are committed to. It's a way of showing them this love, trust, support and commitment. It's also a lot of fun.

So if this is sex at its best, why should you encourage your child to settle for less?

 **Top Tip:** *It's your task to help your child understand that sex is really about the people involved, not the act itself.*

# In the Driving Seat

## How to Help Your Child Take
## Control of Their Decisions

Of course, if it's true that sex is best enjoyed as part of a long-term committed relationship, it makes sense to take care how we handle it *before* such a relationship. So one big question your child may ask is, 'How far should I go before marriage?' And the truth is, there's no easy answer.

It would be handy for every parent to have a relationship checklist they could pass on to their child, detailing just how far it is all right to go in each relationship. For example:

- 'You can kiss, but don't use your tongue'
- 'You can grope, but not to orgasm'
- 'You can fondle breasts, but don't undress'.

Unfortunately, it's not as simple as that. At the end of the day, your child is the only person who can set *their* limits. What's more, as they get older and more responsible, maturing not just sexually but emotionally as well, these limits may change.

That's why you need to ensure that you *don't stop* talking to your child about sex. It's not enough to hand down a few guidelines or commandments and expect them to be followed. Do your best to keep the conversation open. Your child may need your advice (though on their own terms) if they're to keep setting themselves reasonable, responsible and realistic limits.

But if there are no detailed guidelines, there is at least a Golden Rule. There's a story of a rich old woman who lived in a fabulous mansion halfway up a steep mountain. The only access was via a narrow and winding road. When her old chauffeur died, she interviewed three drivers to take his place. She asked each of them in turn just one question: 'How close to the edge could you take me without plunging down the mountain?'

The first replied, 'I could take you to within two feet, but I wouldn't risk taking you any further out than that.'

The second said, 'I'm so good that I could take you to within six inches of the edge and you'd never be in any danger.'

The third was older, wiser and a little more cautious: 'I wouldn't take you anywhere near the edge, madam,' he replied. 'I don't believe in taking unnecessary risks.'

Who got the job? Number Three. It's the same with sex and relationships: it makes sense not to go too 'close to the edge'.

For example, many couples engage in what's technically known as 'heavy petting'. When I was growing up, I thought this was wrestling with a St Bernard! In fact, of course, it's groping on a sofa with your clothes half off, fondling each other's boobs or balls. It can even include oral sex – anything but penetration. In theory, that's where the line is drawn. That's where the cliff edge is. But the thing is, when you've got this far, however resolved you may be not to go further, it's extremely easy to ignore the little voice inside your head telling you to stop ... and end up having full vaginal sex. The experience is so enjoyable you want to get as close as you possibly can to the edge of the cliff without going over. As Woody Allen once said, casual sex may be an empty experience, but as empty experiences go, it's one of the best! However, it takes a huge amount of self-discipline to control that much passion when your hormones are pumping and you're half naked with someone you fancy. So it makes sense to draw a line further back, at a point where you're still in control.

---

 ***Top Tip:*** *You can't set your child's limits for them, but you **can** help them set realistic and responsible limits for themselves.*

---

### 'Let's Talk About Sex'

It's important, therefore, for you to talk things through with your child, and help them set their own personal limits, *before* they ever get into a relationship. Leaving it all to the last minute is a recipe for disaster, because they won't have had time to think it all through and know *why* they've set themselves a limit where they have. As a result, all they'll do is create a rule destined, and almost designed, to be broken.

But it's also important to encourage your child, when they

have a boyfriend or girlfriend, to talk through with *them* what they think the right limits for the physical side of their relationship should be. This might send them both bright purple with embarrassment, of course, and it isn't exactly the height of spontaneous romance – most teenagers are tempted to think that if sex doesn't catch you unawares it's not quite authentic – but it's important for you to encourage them to do it anyway. Firmly agreed ground rules may kill off the illusion that sex 'just happens', but that's not necessarily a bad thing.

What's more, agreed rules will help your child and their boyfriend or girlfriend build trust, which will strengthen their relationship. It will also allow them to enjoy the level of intimacy they *do* share without constantly wondering or worrying about things going any further. If they know that stroking is as far as it goes, they can relax and enjoy it rather than just seeing it as the warm-up act for something more. In the long run, this will help your child see that *foreplay* is something to be savoured in its own right, not something to be rushed through as quickly as humanly possible in the headlong rush to coital climax.

The limits should be what they both feel comfortable with. If one has more conservative limits than the other, *these* are the ones that should be observed. Your child needs to know that it's wrong to force someone to do things they're not ready for, putting undue pressure on them simply because it's what *they* want to do. In other words, arguments like, 'If you really loved me, you'd have sex with me', are nothing but a crude form of emotional blackmail. If someone really loves you, they won't try to make you do anything you're not happy with. If they don't respect your limits, they don't respect you. And if they don't respect you, they don't love you.

**Top Tip:** *Encourage your child to talk their limits through with their boyfriend or girlfriend **before** they're needed.*

## The Be-All-And-End-All?

Agreed limits have one more advantage: they'll encourage your child to explore more in a relationship than merely their boyfriend or girlfriend's body. It may sound strange at first, but in terms of building a fulfilling and lasting relationship, physical beauty is probably the least important aspect! Of course, it's what attracts us initially to another person, but if it doesn't soon give rise to other things, the relationship is doomed to failure. Beauty isn't enough on its own. To prove the point, men with stunningly beautiful wives still have affairs, even if their lover is less attractive than their wife.

Any relationship that's going to last has to be based on more than physical attraction. It's well known that power cuts are peak times for sexual activity, since with the television off some couples find they've forgotten how to talk to one another, and have nothing really left in common except sex. All relationships begin with physical attraction, but if that's *all* they begin with, they're likely to fizzle out quickly. After a few days or weeks admiring or even bonking each other, the couple discover they actually have nothing to *say* to one another.

So encourage your child and their boyfriend or girlfriend to develop some shared interests together, building up an all-round

83

friendship. If they spend all their time locked in a room playing tonsil hockey, they could well be sowing the seeds of disaster. Bimbos and himbos, despite their good looks and athletic physiques, have a limited shelf-life, because no matter how good-looking an individual may be, what's *really* attractive to people is who they are inside. In other words, your child's most important sexual organ isn't their nose, eyes, boobs, butt, penis or vagina. It's their brain. Encourage them to *use* it.

**Top Tip:** *Encourage your child to develop their social skills, not just their kissing style: what makes someone attractive is who they are inside.*

# A Healthy Alternative?

## What If Your Child Is Gay?

'It was never easy for me. I was born a poor black child.'

Nathan Johnson has grown up in an exclusively black, somewhat isolated neighbourhood in Mississippi. One day, his adoring black parents decide the time has finally come for them to tell him the truth: not only is he adopted, but he's also . . . well . . . *white*! As portrayed by Steve Martin in the film *The Jerk*, Nathan doesn't take the news too well. In fact, to be blunt, the bottom drops out of his world. Having grown up thinking of himself as black (he's not exactly blessed in the brains department), he finds it a real struggle coming to terms with the fact that he's a little bit different.

Nathan Johnson is a comic character, and his earth-shattering voyage of self-discovery is played for laughs. But in real life, the discovery that you're 'different' can be anything but funny – as most gay people will tell you. What's more, the time they finally break the news to their mum or dad is one that's rarely filled with laughter. In general, it makes no real difference if parents consider homosexuality to be a valid, acceptable lifestyle or an abominable perversion of nature – their *initial* reaction to the news that their child is gay is one of shock. Even those who've had their suspicions tend to be somewhat bowled over when the moment actually comes.

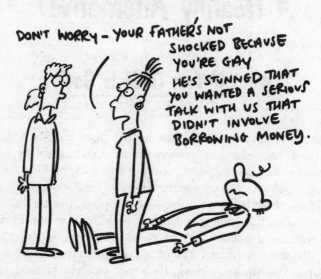

DON'T WORRY - YOUR FATHER'S NOT SHOCKED BECAUSE YOU'RE GAY HE'S STUNNED THAT YOU WANTED A SERIOUS TALK WITH US THAT DIDN'T INVOLVE BORROWING MONEY.

It's understandable, really. After all, most of us develop ideas about what our kids will be like before they're even born. We imagine them growing up to become lawyers, doctors, teachers, homemakers, police officers, plumbers, politicians, pop stars

... the list is endless. We know these are just idle daydreams, of course – as fleeting as many of their *own* early dreams of 'what I'll be when I'm a grown-up'. But some of our preconceptions – the idea that they'll go to college, perhaps, or settle down and have a family – are harder to shake off than others.

In fact, the truth is that however well we get to know them – even if we think we know them inside out – our children still have an amazing ability to surprise us. Most parents are a bit shocked when they discover any side to their child they never knew existed. Whether it's a gift for acting, an aptitude for sport or music, an interest in religion, or a passion for cordon bleu cuisine, the effect is the same: if your child reveals something unexpected about themselves, you'll probably be taken aback. And this is especially true of sexuality.

After all, it's a hotly debated issue. Some people think homosexuality is as 'valid' and 'healthy' a sexual orientation as heterosexuality. Others insist it's a dreadful 'disease' in need of a 'cure'. Theories vary quite considerably as to how a person becomes gay and what, if anything, they can – or should – do about it.

So if your child has told you they're gay – or you're starting to think they *may* be gay – your first reaction is still likely to be one of shock. It may take a few days or weeks for the idea to sink in. This reaction is entirely normal. If they're breaking the news to you, *they'll* have had time to deal with it and prepare themselves for the impact the revelation might have on your relationship – by contrast, *you'll* have had all of about twenty seconds!

**Top Tip:** *If your child tells you they're gay – or you're starting to think they may be gay – your first reaction is likely to be one of shock.*

### 'Was It Something I Said?'

But shock is just the initial stage in a longer process of coming to terms with your child's homosexuality. In many ways, when a parent learns that their child is gay, they go through a series of emotions very similar to those of bereavement:

$$SHOCK \Rightarrow DENIAL \Rightarrow PAIN \Rightarrow ACCEPTANCE$$

So if your first reaction is one of shock, your second is likely to be denial or disbelief. 'Are you sure?'

A small number of gay people initially tell a friend or parent they're gay in part as a way of finding out if it still rings true once they've said it. But don't hold your breath, hoping your child will have a change of heart, because the vast majority of gay people don't risk their parents' rejection unless they're 99 per cent sure it's true. They're more likely to tell you because you're important to them and they need the reassurance that comes from knowing you still love them. It's not easy to be gay. It may no longer be a crime, as it was at the turn of the twentieth century, but there's still a lot of stigma attached to the label 'homosexual'. In fact, your child will almost certainly have found it a Herculean effort, several months in the planning, just to pluck up the courage to tell you about it!

The third stage in the process of coming to terms with your child's homosexuality isn't so much pain as *puzzlement* and *guilt*. Most parents are full of questions when they find out their child is gay. 'Where did this come from? Why me? Why *them*? Was it something I said? Did I do something wrong? Did they get it from me? What about grandchildren?'

When they start coming to terms with the situation, most parents of a gay child – whether they think homosexuality is something to be valued or vilified – have to deal with feelings of guilt. There's a deep down, irrational fear that something they said or did, or something lurking in their DNA, was responsible for their child's sexuality – for giving them, at the very least, an uphill struggle for social acceptance. But as powerful as these guilt feelings are, they're misplaced. No one knows just what makes one person gay and another person not. It's still something of a scientific mystery. But what *is* clear from all the research done into the causes of homosexuality (and heterosexuality) is that there's no simple explanation.

In other words, if you could fast-rewind back through your child's life, as if it were all on video tape, you'd never be able to find anything you said or did – or failed to say or do – that was *entirely responsible* for making them gay. What's more, homo-sexuality can't be 'caught' from a parent as if it were a disease: almost all gay people come from exclusively *hetero*sexual homes. And you can't even attribute your child's homosexuality to the genes they inherited from you. The truth is that it's *much* more complicated than that.

> **Top Tip:** Don't be tempted to think your child is gay just because of something you may have said or done – the causes are much more complicated than that.

## All Change?

For a long time, both medical and public opinion saw homosexuality as a wilful, stubborn and evil practice that had to be dealt with severely by a decent, civilised society. But at the start of the twentieth century, when the science of psychology was in its infancy, this kind of thinking began to change. Instead, doctors and psychologists began to see it as a form of illness that could be treated – at least in theory. Being gay was seen as a 'perversion' of the 'normal' sex drive, and homosexuals were classified as 'deviants'. This remained true until 1973, when both the American Psychiatric Association and the World Health Organisation officially removed homosexuality from their lists of 'psychiatric disorders'.

Contrary to what some people believe, this change in medical opinion wasn't a result of the new 'permissive' society – it came because doctors started to get a better understanding of what *type* of person was gay. Back in the 1950s, the three main medical explanations for the cause of homosexuality – hormones, heredity and the home environment – all took it for granted that gay people were psychologically *ab*normal. The reason for this is simple: these explanations were devised by doctors and psychiatrists who based their opinions on what their gay patients were telling them. But, of course, by definition, these patients were people who were seeking help because they felt that homosexuality *was* abnormal.

By the 1970s, it was becoming clear that, except for their sexual orientation, gay people are *exactly* like heterosexual people. Effeminate men and 'butch' women may be what we first think of when we hear the word 'homosexual', but that's far from being the whole story. Homosexuality isn't linked to how 'feminine' or 'masculine' a person seems to be. It's as misguided to assume that all gay men are as 'feminine' as Julian Clary (or that all effeminate men are gay) as it is to think that all heterosexual men are as macho as Arnold Schwarzeneggar (or that all macho men are heterosexual)!

In other words, homosexuality has nothing whatsoever to do with what makes us physically more 'masculine' or 'feminine': hormone levels. People aren't gay because they have too little of their own sex hormone or too much of the opposite hormone. Medically speaking, gay men and women are totally normal. In fact, the truth is that we *all* have *both* male hormones (such as testosterone) *and* female hormones (oestrogens). Some men have a more 'feminine' appearance because their body produces too much oestrogen or too little testosterone. Similarly, some women appear more 'masculine' than normal because their body produces too much testosterone or too little oestrogen. But this isn't at all linked to homosexuality. Hormone imbalance can affect *appearance*, but there's no evidence to prove that 'effeminate' or 'masculine' *behaviour* is caused by a lack of appropriate sex hormones.

Quite the opposite, actually. Some people have a hormone

91

deficiency caused by having an odd number of chromosomes: dense coils of DNA, each containing thousands of genes. Almost every cell in your body has forty-six chromosomes, two of which – 'X' (female) and 'Y' (male) – determine your gender. Women normally have two X chromosomes and men have an X and a Y. But women with Turner's Syndrome only have *one* X chromosome, and need regular oestrogen injections from puberty onwards in order to grow breasts and menstruate. If homosexuality were caused by a hormone imbalance, you'd expect women with Turner's Syndrome who aren't given extra hormones to be gay. In fact, they tend to be uninterested in sex altogether. What's more, rather than behaving in a more masculine way, women with Turner's Syndrome are routinely more feminine. And it's a similar story for men with Klinefelter's Syndrome, who have two X chromosomes as well as the normal Y. Without testosterone injections, they may *look* more feminine, but they're no different to other men in terms of their *behaviour* or sexual orientation.

In other words, if you have a son who's more interested in cooking than the Cup Final, or a daughter who'd rather play with barbells than Barbie dolls, don't jump to the hasty conclusion they must be gay, or march them off to the GP. And if your otherwise 'normal' child calmly informs you they *are* gay, don't expect them to become someone or something else overnight. Some gay people naturally fit traditional stereotypes, but the vast majority don't. Your child will be exactly the same person they were *before* they told you.

**Top Tip:** *Only a few gay people fit the stereo-types, so don't expect your child to turn into someone different just because they're gay.*

## A Decent Pair of Genes . . .

But if homosexuality isn't in the hormones, what does cause it? At first glance, there appear to be just two 'prime suspects': *heredity* ('nature') and the *home environment* ('nurture'). Is one of these responsible?

As part of the recent ongoing work to map the whole of the human 'genome' – working out what every strand of DNA in the body does – some scientists claim to have discovered a 'gay gene'. There is, they suggest, a sequence of DNA found in many gay people, but not heterosexual people, which strongly points to the idea that homosexual orientation has its basis in human genetics. Many gay groups have seized on the discovery as clear proof that gay people can't help being gay, and shouldn't try – they're gay because their genes *make* them that way. Their DNA *predetermines* them to be homosexual.

But whilst it's attractive to many gay people, this theory doesn't actually hold water. The cracks become clear when you look at studies done on identical twins. Identical twins are very important to geneticists, since every scrap of their DNA is exactly the same. In other words, any differences between them in behaviour or personality can't be a result of their genes because their genes are *identical*. They can only be a result of the twins

93

having had different experiences or having made slightly different decisions. If being gay were all part and parcel of a person's genes, then identical twins should have identical sexual orientation. Either *both* of them should be gay, or *neither* of them should be. The problem is, this just isn't the case. Some identical twins have different sexual orientations: one is gay, one isn't.

But there's another crack in the theory, and it comes from the science of genetics itself. A single gene or gene group can certainly *predetermine* simple things like height, hair colour, skin colour or weight bracket. Genes can even go a long way toward *shaping* someone's personality, which is why identical twins who have for one reason or another been raised apart can be very similar in temperament. But genes can't predetermine personality, which is why identical twins raised apart will also have lots of differences in their character.

To put it bluntly, human behaviour is too complex to be preset like a car radio or passed on in the genes. It's obvious, really: if behaviour were predetermined by genes, schools and parents wouldn't need to teach children how to behave. You wouldn't need to tell your child about wise and responsible sexual behaviour (whatever their orientation) – the genes would do it automatically. Of course, as a mum or dad, you know only too well that behaviour is something children need to *learn*. And sexual behaviour is perhaps the most complex of all. It's not preset by DNA, even if genes do give people a nudge in one direction or another.

The truth of this became all too obvious recently to the staff of a South African game reserve when a group of young male elephants became out of control, attacking tourists and trying to mate with or kill the park's female rhinos. One elephant even killed the professional hunter who was sent to shoot it! As they observed the delinquent elephants over a period of three years, the park's experts reached a startling conclusion: they were misbehaving because their mothers hadn't been around to teach them how to behave properly. Once they'd been weaned, the staff had naturally assumed it was safe to separate the young elephants from their mums, moving them to different game reserves. But the result of this policy was catastrophic: despite having a perfect set of genes, the young elephants still didn't know how to behave because they'd never been *taught* how to behave.

So your child's DNA didn't *predetermine* that they should be gay. Genes can play a very big part, but they can't make it an entirely done deal. They just don't have that kind of control on anything as complicated as sexual orientation and behaviour.

> **Top Tip:** *Your child's DNA may have played an important part in their becoming gay, but by themselves genes are only half the story.*

## Home, Sweet Home

So if 'nature' isn't responsible, what about 'nurture'? The third explanation for the cause of homosexuality popular in the 1950s, besides hormones and heredity, was concerned with a child's home environment. In particular, some doctors and psychiatrists were convinced that gay men (they didn't do much research into gay women) were basically 'mother's boys'.

In this, they were echoing a view expressed as long ago as 1730 in a book called *Plain Reasons for the Growth of Sodomy in England*, which argued that homosexuality was a danger to the future health of the British Empire, and attacked the way in which young boys were 'mollycoddled' and sent to kindergartens run by women!

By the 1950s, this view had become much more refined: boys with domineering mothers and weak fathers, some doctors argued, grew up without a strong male influence and didn't know how to be 'real men'. As a result, they were often attacked as 'sissies' and came to have a negative view of the traditional 'masculine' role in both society and sex. Lacking self-confidence, and hampered by a crushing sense of inferiority, they made little headway with girls, turning instead to like-minded boys. Today, as it becomes increasingly clear that very few gay men are 'mother's boys', the value of this theory as an explanation for the causes of homosexuality is practically zero.

The truth is, gay men and women grow up in home environments every bit as varied and 'ordinary' as heterosexual men and women. There's nothing about a gay person's home life or background that can be singled out as having caused their sexual orientation. There's no common thread linking the home environment and upbringing of all homosexual people. So far as we know, all cultures throughout history have included gay people, though attitudes to them have varied considerably. The Greeks and Romans, for example, had a positive approach to male homosexual activity – though they had strict rules about who could do what with whom – and our word for a homosexual woman, 'lesbian', is derived from the Greek island of Lesbos, where the woman poet Sappho, writing in 600 BC, is said to have noted same-sex love between women. In none of these cultures is there an identifiable set of circumstances that can be demonstrated to produce homosexual orientation in a child.

In fact, the evidence suggests just the opposite. Some ancient cultures – like those of New Guinea and Australia, for example – saw homosexual activity as a 'stage' all males went through between puberty and marriage – a kind of 'rite of passage'. But whilst these societies may have expected that all boys of a certain age should *act* in a homosexual way, this did nothing to alter their fundamental sexual orientation. When this 'homosexual' period was over, the majority had exclusively *heterosexual* relationships. In other words, even this kind of 'social conditioning' couldn't make 'straight' people gay or gay people 'straight'. Human behaviour and sexuality is much more complicated than that.

So don't imagine that something you've done or will do – or haven't done or might fail to do at some time in the future – is solely responsible for altering your child's basic sexual orientation. In fact, scientists have now largely abandoned the idea that there's a single stand-alone cause for homosexuality. Instead, the most plausible explanation is that people become homosexual or heterosexual (or bisexual, attracted to either gender) through a combination of different factors, all interwoven and none uniquely responsible.

 ***Top Tip:*** *DNA and domestic environment combine to determine if a child is gay or not, so don't look for one, simple cause.*

## 'My Heart's Just Not in It!'

Of course, one result of there being no simple cause of homosexuality is that there's also no simple way to prevent a person being gay. This comes as unwelcome news for some parents, who are worried that their child is, or might be, gay and desperately want them *not* to be. Some parents are convinced that homosexuality is a 'perversion', and want their child to be free of it. Others have no moral objection, but don't want them to have to go through the ordeal of being gay in a world where homosexuality isn't universally accepted.

But the fact is, you can't *make* your child *hetero*sexual – any more than you can *make* them *homo*sexual. Though our choices – both big decisions and seemingly insignificant ones – help shape who we are just as much as our genes and our environment, being gay isn't something over which gay people feel they have a choice. After all, who in their right mind would *choose* to expose themselves to the emotional trauma and social discrimination that inevitably seem to accompany being gay in this day and age?

In fact, most gay people are *aware* of their sexuality by the age of about five or six, even if it then takes them another decade to *recognise* it for what it is, and perhaps even another decade still to *reveal* it. At five or six, most of us can't even spell 'sex', let alone make conscious decisions about anything as complex as sexual orientation. In other words, the vast majority of gay children don't *choose* to be homosexual any more than heterosexual children *choose* to be heterosexual. It's not *their* decision any more than it is *yours*.

But if they can't choose it, ninety-nine times out of a hundred they can't change it either. In the past, doctors who attempted to 'cure' homosexuality often prescribed a heterosexual relationship as an effective remedy. In Ian Fleming's James Bond adventure, *Goldfinger*, lesbian bad girl Pussy Galore is magically transformed into a card-carrying heterosexual after just one night with 007! In real life, however, all that really changed through such 'cures' was *action*, not *orientation*. As a result, the 'cure' often proved as bad as, if not worse than, the 'disease'. Exclusively gay men and women found themselves trapped in loveless marriages, going through the motions with a partner they didn't really find attractive. And bisexual men and women found themselves acting on their heterosexual feelings and desires, pretending that the homosexual feelings and desires they also had were 'dealt with' when they'd actually just been swept under the carpet.

If your child is *uncomfortable* with their sexuality, ask your family doctor to put you in touch with someone they can talk to about it – a qualified professional who will help them slowly work through the issues. But if they've come to terms with being gay by themselves, don't try to change them or talk them out of it – you'll only succeed in driving a wedge between the two of you, damaging your relationship and destroying any basis of trust. To put it simply, the more you try and change them, the more you send them the message that you don't love them the way they are, and that's a recipe for nothing short of disaster.

---

 **Top Tip:** *Whatever your moral views may be, don't try to change your child's sexuality – they'll think you don't love them the way they are.*

---

## 'Give Me Your Unconditional Love'

In the film *Dead Poets Society*, Neil Perry's dad pushes him to become a doctor. It's not that he particularly wants Neil to go into medicine – he just wants him to have something to fall back on, whatever happens. He carefully plans the first twenty-five years of Neil's life, keeping a firm grip on everything he does. And to make him focus on his studies, he bans Neil from all out-of-school activities. But Neil himself has other ideas, and when he secretly auditions for a local production of *A Midsummer Night's Dream*, landing a lead role, he knows he's found what he wants to do with his life: become an actor. When Mr Perry finds out, he's livid. He loves Neil immensely, but he's convinced he'll be jeopardising his future security and happiness if he doesn't at least qualify as a doctor. So he decides to take him out of his strict, regimented school and send him to an even stricter and more regimented one.

Tragically, the message this sends Neil is that his dad can only love him on the condition that he stops being himself. After all, acting is what makes him feel most alive, and most comfortable with who he is. If his dad can't love him as an actor, Neil concludes, he can't love him at all – only the respectable, presentable, medical version he feels Neil should be. And Neil can't live with this, because it isn't true to what he feels is his real personality. Spiralling into depression, he ends his own life with his father's gun.

If your child is a teenager – which is when many gay people recognise their sexuality for what it is – they're already in the middle of one of the most vulnerable times of their life. If they're also coming to terms with being gay, they'll probably be even more vulnerable. They may not be suicidal, of course, but they'll still be hesitant, unsure of themselves and still struggling with the full implications of their revelation.

The stigma attached to being gay, added to the strong sense of isolation that comes from knowing you're different to most of your friends, can be a volatile mix in a teenager. Most teenagers feel the need to be exactly the same as their friends – the feeling of acceptance it gives them helps them to develop a proper sense of self-worth. If your child is gay, they'll instinctively know that their friends will find it hard to accept them, so they'll look for that sense of acceptance from somewhere else – and like it or not, that somewhere else is *you*.

Every child needs to know that their mum and/or dad loves them unconditionally, with no strings attached. They need to feel supported, cherished, welcomed, accepted, encouraged, and as important to *themselves* as they are to *you*. They need to know that wherever they go in life, whatever they do and however they turn out, you'll always love them. Even when you disapprove of what they do – even when you think they're a real 'prodigal son' – you'll never judge them or put conditions on your love for them. Even when you have to point out their mistakes or punish them, you'll do so in such a way that they understand you couldn't stop loving them if you tried. They need to know you love them to bits for who they are, not what they do or don't do. Without this unconditional love, your child's emotions can't develop properly.

This doesn't stop being true just because a child is gay. In fact, if anything, it becomes even more important, as gay people are open to so much hostility and negative comment from the world around them. If your child has told you they're gay, you can be sure they haven't done so just to keep you up-to-date on their private life – they're looking for the reassurance and affirmation that only you, as their mum or dad, can give them.

Discovering and exploring your sexuality is hard enough at the best of times, whether you're homosexual or heterosexual. It's always full of risk and fraught with tension. It's easy to get hurt and make mistakes. It's easy to get so carried away by the moment that you lose track of the big picture and act irresponsibly. It's easy to lose sight of your importance and imagine you're not worth anything. Bouncing back from these kinds of mistakes and misconceptions is a lot easier with the unconditional love and support of a parent.

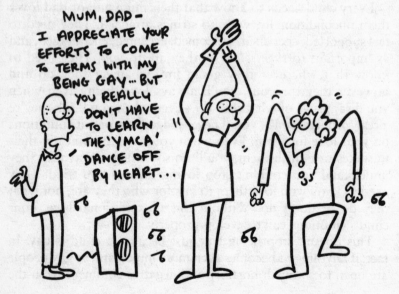

MUM, DAD – I APPRECIATE YOUR EFFORTS TO COME TO TERMS WITH MY BEING GAY... BUT YOU REALLY DON'T HAVE TO LEARN THE 'YMCA' DANCE OFF BY HEART...

So above all, whatever your personal views on homosexuality may be, try to ensure they never blind you to the vital importance of loving your child unconditionally. You may have a tough time coming to terms with it – most parents do. You may have moral objections to your son or daughter being gay. But your job as a parent isn't to sort through their sexuality or make their sexual choices *for* them – it's to give them the love and support they need as they do this for *themselves*.

 **Top Tip:** *What your child needs from you is **unconditional love** as they sort through their sexuality and make their own sexual choices.*

# 'Just Our Little Secret'

## How to Talk to Your Child
## about Sexual Abuse

When the prestigious ocean liner company White Star launched the Royal Mail Steamer *Titanic* in April 1912, it was confident it had built not just the largest passenger vessel in the world, but also the safest. Her riveted steel, double-bottomed construction, along with her electrically operated water-tight compartments, led the press to go as far as dubbing her 'unsinkable'. But five days into her maiden voyage to New York, the *Titanic* hit an iceberg. The rest, as they say, is history. Never again would any shipbuilder be so cavalier. Never again would they dare to believe that the unthinkable could never happen to them.

For most of us, the idea that our child might be raped or abused is just as unthinkable. It's such an appalling prospect that we put it right out of our minds, unable – or unwilling – to see it as a real possibility. Sexual abuse is always something that happens to *other people's* children, not *our own*. But to adopt this approach is to invite potential disaster, in the same way that White Star's overconfident attitude led to the tragic loss of the *Titanic*.

Talking to your child about the risk of sexual abuse isn't just wise, it's *essential*. We need to take the possible threat of harm seriously enough to ensure that we take sufficient safety precautions, but without overreacting. It's important for us to keep things in perspective, steering a middle course between complacency and paranoia. We mustn't let our fears get in the way of our child's dreams, allowing ourselves to get so worked up about the potential danger of abuse that we put them under 24-hour surveillance or lock them indoors for life. When the *Titanic* sank, rather than putting an end to all transcontinental shipping, the government tightened up the safety precautions. In the same way, airline companies don't close down their businesses simply because they know it's possible for one of their planes to crash – instead, they take careful precautions and give all passengers safety demonstrations before every flight. Their aim is simple: not to frighten the passengers or cabin crew out of their wits, but to make sure they know what to do in case the 'unthinkable' happens and they have to make an emergency landing.

 **Top Tip:** *Without overreacting, it's important to face the possibility that your child could be harmed. Ignorance is a recipe for potential disaster.*

## One in a Million?

Child sexual abuse is alarmingly common. In the US, where lots of research has been done into the frequency of sexual abuse, conservative estimates by experts indicate that about one in five children has experienced some form of sexual abuse by the time they reach their eighteenth birthday – either 'abuse' as a child, or 'harassment' or 'rape' (including so-called 'date-rape') as an adolescent. Research in the UK puts this figure much lower, at about one in ten children (one in eight girls, one in twelve boys), but a number of factors – including the famous 'British reserve' – may be responsible for less harm being reported here than in America. At any rate, one in ten is far from being an isolated phenomenon.

To put it in even starker terms, you probably know several people who were sexually harmed as children. Of course, they don't wear badges advertising the fact, and don't have 'victim' tattooed across their forehead, so the chances are you just don't know they were harmed. After all, it's not something we generally talk about.

But *that's* the problem. Because we don't talk about it, we create a culture of silence round the issue. We make it a taboo subject. It's a catch-22. Because it's such a hard subject to talk about, we tend not to talk about it. But because we tend not to talk about it, it remains a hard subject to talk about. What's more, not talking about it keeps us misinformed, which in turn stops us from appreciating just how vitally important it is *to* talk about it. So the silence continues, the ignorance continues and the harm continues.

Ignorance *isn't* bliss. Of course we don't want to scare our children – or ourselves – into distrusting everyone they know. After all, 90 per cent of children are *not* harmed. But if we don't inform them sufficiently about *their* rights and *other people's* wrongs, we're leaving them unprepared to deal with the lies an abuser might tell them. Knowledge is power: by telling your child about the possible threat of harm, you'll be empowering them to protect themselves from that threat if it ever arises.

**Top Tip:** *However old they are, your child needs to know the truth about sexual abuse for their own protection.*

### Once Upon a Time . . .

Harm can range from touching a child's genitals or other parts of their body with the aim of producing sexual excitement in the person doing the touching, to inserting a penis or some other object into a child's anus or vagina. It doesn't have to involve anyone reaching orgasm and it doesn't have to involve nudity. Forcing a child to read or watch sexually explicit material is also a form of harm – it too involves exploiting a child for sexual satisfaction. Legally, a 'child' is defined as anyone unable to give informed consent to sex – at the time of writing, that means under eighteen for male same-sex encounters and under sixteen for opposite-sex ones.

Against the background of all the misunderstandings people have about sexual abuse, five facts deserve special mention because they're so commonly overlooked.

**1. Your child is most at risk from someone they know.** When a convicted paedophile was released from prison to a halfway-house in their area, local residents took their protest to the streets, afraid for their children's safety. But the fear of 'stranger danger' blinded them to the truth that the greatest risk to their children's safety came from closer to home. Two-thirds of all harm is done by someone a child knows and trusts. Far from being an old man in a raincoat, the typical person who harms a child is a parent, brother, sister, uncle, aunt, grandparent, friend, babysitter, teacher, youth worker – someone in a position of trust who spends time alone with children. Of course, it's vital not to blow things out of proportion: most of the people your child knows and trusts – probably *all* of them – wouldn't dream of harming them. But if your child is among the one in ten who are harmed, they're twice as likely to be harmed by someone they're in regular contact with than by the stereotypical paedophile.

**2. People who harm children seem very ordinary.** In 1960, after a fifteen year search, Israeli intelligence captured Adolf Eichmann, the man responsible for arranging the murder of six million Jews in the Holocaust. His trial made news around the world, but what shocked people most was how *ordinary* he was. Don't be tempted to think you could spot an abuser at thirty paces. There's more to an abuser than just their abuse – in other respects they *seem* normal because in other respects that's exactly what they *are*. Most adults who harm children

109

hide their abusive streak as thoroughly as they hide the abuse. And though many were themselves victims as a child (though it's important to point out that most victims *don't* go on to harm children themselves), they still tend to convince themselves they're not doing anything wrong. Many even think their victims actually enjoy the experience.

**3. Men and women harm children.** Though girls are twice as likely to be harmed as boys, it is thought that between 80 and 95 per cent of all sexual abuse cases involve a male abuser. Nevertheless, it would be wrong to think that women *don't* harm children, or that when they do they only harm girls. Not only are some women abusers themselves, others are passive participants in their husband or partner's abuse, allowing it to happen by refusing to see, or admit, what's really going on.

**4. Many men who harm boys are heterosexual, and may even be married.** It used to be said that men who harmed boys were gay, but the truth is that much same-gender harm is done by *heterosexual* people. (In fact, as the word suggests, the stereotypical 'paedophile' tends to be sexually attracted to *children*, not adults at all.) The truth is that *sexual abuse is about power, not sex*. Many married abusers treat their spouse in the same harmful way they treat children – the common thread is the intoxicating sense of power it gives them. Sexual orientation actually plays almost no part in abuse – a victim's gender is far less important than their vulnerability, because abuse is basically a form of sexual bullying.

**5. Sexual abuse is a well-kept secret.** Many parents assume they'd know if their child was being harmed – they know their child well enough to pick up on any change in their behaviour. But the problem is that all the 'classic' warning signs –

chronically low self-esteem, inappropriate sexual behaviour or knowledge, disruptive activity, an inability to concentrate, fear of intimacy, physical markers such as bruising, etc. – can be the result of a great many things *other than* sexual abuse. What's more, through a mix of fear, guilt and shame, your child is unlikely to volunteer any information about it.

 **Top Tip:** *Your child* isn't *immune from the risk of harm, and sadly the biggest threat is likely to come from someone they know and trust.*

## The Guilty Party

All adults exert power over children, and the closer and more trusted an adult is, the more power they have. There's nothing wrong with this. In fact, it's healthy. Parents and schools would be lost without it – we rely on the power and authority we wield over our children to get them to do everything from finishing their homework and being polite to washing behind their ears and staying away from naked flames. But power must always be used in a responsible way. As parents, we're responsible for ensuring that our children grow up safe and sound to make their own wise choices in life.

Sexual abuse – causing a child what's now referred to as 'significant harm' – involves the use of *power without responsibility*. Though it involves sex, it's actually about unscrupulous bullies exerting power for their own selfish gain. They ignore

111

their responsibility to use this power for a child's good. Sometimes this involves the use of brute force, but more often than not it involves far subtler forms of *persuasion*. As a result, some parents, most abusers and almost all victims can wonder just who's to blame. Does the victim share in the guilt? Did they give their consent? Are they in part responsible for the harm?

The answer to these questions is an unequivocal **no,** for two reasons.

The first reason is simple: no child under sixteen is legally *entitled* to give consent to sex, so the harm *can't* happen with their consent. And why can't children legally give consent? Because society doesn't think they're emotionally or mentally responsible or mature enough to make that kind of decision yet. The burden of responsibility therefore rests with the adult. In other words, when an adult harms a child, *they alone* are responsible. Legally and morally, the child is in no way to blame.

After months of therapy, Paul – a man who had harmed his own daughter – was still trying to justify his actions to both his wife and his therapist. 'Cindy was running around with only a towel on,' he explained, 'giving me the eye, you know the way she does.' With a hint of desperation, he added, 'I'm not the only one to blame for what happened.'

'But Paul,' the wife replied, 'Cindy was only seven years old!'

The second reason is more complicated: children are usually eager to please and highly impressionable. This gives adults considerable power over them. Again, this isn't bad – we rely on it to teach them right from wrong, enabling them to make good choices in later life. But in cases of harm, this power is *ab*used: a child's eagerness to please is hijacked and taken advantage of for someone else's selfish gain.

When ten-year-old Billy was sent to stay with his aunt for a few days, he could barely contain his excitement. He loved his aunt, and they had always got on well. But on his first night, rather than tucking him into bed, she started to unbutton his pyjamas. In spite of her soothing words, he *knew* the way she was touching him was wrong, and desperately wanted her to stop. At the same time, he loved his aunt and didn't want to upset her. He was afraid that if he said no, she'd stop loving him. In the end, he 'let' her harm him only because he didn't know how to make it stop without losing her love. His desire for approval and his eagerness to please – natural childhood qualities – conspired against him because, and *only* because, they were hijacked by his aunt. For all his subsequent guilt feelings, Billy wasn't in any way to blame for the harm. His aunt was.

 **Top Tip:** *Harm is an abuse of **power** even more than it's an abuse of sex – never let a child feel they're at all to blame. They're not.*

## The Best Defence

The first line of defence is always to take a good hard look at the different environments and activities your child is involved in outside the home. As much as possible, your goal should be to minimise the risk of an adult harming them through a combination of taking common-sense precautions and creating safe protective environments for them.

For example, your child will be safer if you:

- always take and fetch them from organised activities, or ask a trusted friend or relative to do this for you
- never leave them as the last one to be collected from outside activities
- try and be there to watch if they're playing sports or taking part in any outside activity
- encourage them to play at your house, and invite their friends, especially if they have a space (bedroom, playroom, corner of the dining room, etc.) that's theirs
- try to know where they are at all times
- make sure they know your phone number, and give them a phone card or change for a pay phone (or a mobile phone if they're older) so they can always contact you if they're in trouble or need to tell you where they are
- remain vigilant if an adult is showing them special attention
- notice if they have any unexplained gifts or money
- make sure that every organisation your child comes into contact with has an adequate child protection policy. This should ensure that all staff are trained in child protection, and that they were thoroughly interviewed when they were hired and their background was properly checked. It should also guarantee there are *always* two members of staff supervising children, so no one is ever given a chance to be alone with your child.

You don't need to turn your home into Fort Knox or get M15 to accompany your ten-year-old son and his friends every time they go down to the park for a game of football, but you do need to take *sensible* precautions.

 **Top Tip:** *The best way to prevent anyone harming your child is to create protective environments for them and take sensible precautions.*

## Home and Away

But since you can't always control your child's environment, it's also vital to tell them the facts about harm, and help them develop the self-confidence to say no to any improper advance – whether it's by someone they know or someone they've never met before.

### Danger from a Stranger

When it comes to 'stranger danger', it's important to adopt a twofold approach:

- **Yell-Run-Tell.** Teach your child the Kidscape Yell-Run-Tell rule: **yell** 'No!' loudly, **run** to somewhere safe (where others are around) and **tell** an adult what's happened
- **Don't Talk to Strangers.** Teach your child *not* to talk to, go with or accept gifts from strangers, whatever they say.

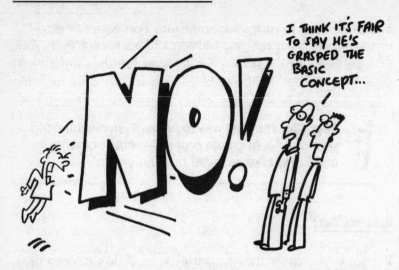

## Danger from Someone They Know

As we've seen, however, the biggest threat to your child doesn't come from strangers – it comes from people they know and trust. So as well as the twofold approach to strangers, you'll also need to teach them the following threefold approach to coping with the threat of harm from someone they know.

- **Know Your Rights.** Your child's basic right *not* to be harmed is, of course, enshrined in law. But rights don't always translate into reality. Abusers make victims feel they're not in control, and don't have a right to say no. So it's crucial for you to teach your child that they have a *right* not to be sexually harmed. Anyone trying to touch them in an inappropriate way – one that makes them feel uncomfortable –

is therefore in the *wrong*. Children instinctively know that harm is wrong, of course, but the ability to convince them otherwise is part of the power held by an abuser, especially one they trust. So the more you teach your child that they have a right to what goes on in relation to their own body – a right to say no at *any* time – the more you'll be able to protect them by helping them to see that they're in the right and the abuser is in the wrong.

- **Know Your Limits.** Of course, knowing your rights doesn't always mean that the harm will stop. As a parent, the last thing you want to do is give your child the idea that they *shouldn't* resist an abuser's advances. On the contrary, you want them to yell, scream, push, shove, kick, bite ... whatever they can to prevent the harm from happening. But sexual abuse is a crime of power – a mixture of brute force, intimidation and emotional blackmail – and sometimes your child will simply be over*powered*. It's vital to explain this possibility to them when you tell them about their rights and saying no. Otherwise, if they *are* overpowered, they may feel they *should* have been able to stop it. And if this happens, not only will they feel partly to blame, they may be so ashamed of what they see as their 'failure' that they're too afraid to tell you about it.

- **Know You're Loved.** Though physical force is involved in harm, it rarely plays as big a role as *emotional* pressure. Most adults have a hard time coming to terms with being rejected by someone they love, whether it's a parent, partner or peer. Children, whose self-worth is still developing, often find the threat of rejection overwhelming. This is what gives an abuser their power. So helping your child realise their true worth – letting them know how much you love them – will give them the self-confidence to say no, and the self-esteem to cope even if resistance is futile. The more they know you love them unconditionally, the less dependent they'll be on an abuser's love and approval.

The golden rule, of course, is to instil into your child the paramount importance of **telling you** about *anyone* who tries to make inappropriate advances to them or touch them in a way that makes them feel uncomfortable. Make sure they know the difference between a 'good' secret (what they're getting you for Christmas) and the kind of 'bad' secret that abusers insist their victims keep. Above all, ensure the communication channels stay open between you and your child, whether they're four or fourteen (or forty).

In addition, it's important to bear two things in mind. First, no matter how old your child is, it's never too late to teach them these 'rules'. Harm doesn't stop just because they reach the age of consent – we just give it different names, such as rape or sexual harassment. Second, it's not just adults who harm – sometimes it's carried out by one child on another. One third of all cautions and convictions for sexual offences in England and Wales involve someone less than twenty-one years of age. Brothers, sisters, cousins, older friends: anyone who wields any kind of power or influence over your child could potentially abuse them if they had the intention and the opportunity. This isn't 'innocent experimentation' or something they'll grow out of – it needs to be treated very seriously. Adolescents who harm children will need help if the pattern isn't to become ingrained, and the harm will be no less real or painful for your child simply because it was carried out by someone who's not yet a fully grown adult.

---

> **Top Tip:** *To help protect your child from harm,* **help** *them to see how valuable they are,* **teach** *them their right to say no and* **encourage** *them to tell you about anyone who makes them feel uncomfortable.*

---

## Help!

But what if your child has already been harmed, and it feels more like a case of trying to close the stable door after the horse has bolted? What then?

The first thing to do if your child tells you they've been harmed is *believe them*. It's rare for a child to make up stories of something as serious as abuse, though when it does happen the consequences for the person accused are devastating and long-lasting. But even if their claim strikes you as unbelievable – especially if it involves someone you know and trust, perhaps even a partner or sibling – your concern as a mum or dad *must* be for your child. The risk involved in believing them – even if they've got a track record of bending the truth a bit – is much, much less than the risk involved in *not* believing them.

Having believed them, and made it clear you believe them, there are three further things for you to do: **stop, look** and **listen**.

119

**Stop.** If there's even a chance that the harm is still going on (and there's some evidence to suggest that children are wary about admitting that harm is continuing), it's imperative for you to make sure that the right steps are taken to stop it. Where there's an immediate threat to life, or in cases where physical evidence (such as semen) may still be present in or on your child, the first people to contact are the police. In most cases, however, it's best to get in touch with your local Social Services Child Protection Team. They're used to dealing with instances of harm, and they'll generally be calm, collected and thorough. Most of the time, they'll make a detailed investigation of everything before taking any necessary action, talking to your child, to you, your partner if you have one, the alleged abuser and any other people (e.g. teachers, youth leader) who can shed light on things. Don't worry about them trying to take your child away from you – under the terms of the 1989 Children Act, Social Services don't have the legal power to remove a child from their parents unless they can prove it would be dangerous to leave them there. In other words, your local authority is *only* allowed to remove your child from you if you or your partner is the one committing the abuse, and there's a clear risk of the harm continuing if they remain at home.

You may be a little cautious about getting Social Services involved. Is it really necessary? The answer is emphatically *yes*. For one thing, your child won't have told you about the harm purely for your information. They'll want help. They'll want it stopped, and Social Services (together with the police) are the people with the power and responsibility to make that happen. For another, more than just *your* child's welfare may be at stake. Though some abusers only ever harm one child or commit sexual offences during only one period of their life, most will harm other children if given the chance. You can't afford to ignore this, however reluctant you may be to 'go public'.

**Look.** Once the harm has been stopped and the abuser is being dealt with, it's time to take a careful look at the damage. Children who've been harmed usually feel dirty, guilty, worthless and unlovable because they've been personally violated. Their most intimate form of expressing affection has been hijacked by someone else for their selfish pleasure. Sex is meaningful only when you positively choose to do it, and for people who've suffered rape or abuse, it can be a long and painful journey to recover this feeling of choice. You'll have to work very hard to reassure them that:

- you love them, with no strings attached
- they're immensely valuable as a person
- you don't judge or condemn them for what's happened
- they're in no way responsible for what's happened
- they're not blemished or marked out for life
- they can still live a happy and fruitful life
- what they've experienced is not sex, but abuse
- they can still find love, and find it wonderful.

It may be helpful to draw a line under the past, removing them from the kind of activity in which they experienced the abuse. Don't be surprised by any seemingly 'irrational' fears and flashbacks connected to it. Harm is not something from which a child will just 'bounce back', however bright and bonny they may appear to be on the surface. Most victims take *years* to come to terms with the emotional impact of their ordeal. Some

121

experience further problems at strategic times of their life like puberty or marriage. You'll have to repeat your affirmative message to them time and time again, giving them evidence over many years of how special they are and how much you love them. They need to hear this even more often than they need(ed) to hear a bedtime story, so get used to *saying* it, *meaning* it, and having them *disbelieve* it on a very regular basis.

**Listen.** It's not good for your child to bottle everything up inside. They'll need to talk to someone who's been professionally trained to understand what they've been through and help them come to terms with it. Your GP or Social Services should be able to refer you to someone qualified in this area. (If you haven't reported the matter to Social Services, it's worth bearing in mind that whilst doctors and therapists – and even clergy – aren't legally obliged to report cases of significant harm, most are bound by a code of ethics that give them no choice but to do so.)

It's not a sign of weakness to seek help. It will be scary and probably very painful for your child to talk about what's happened to them but it's the *only* way for them to be free of it and begin again. You'll play a vital part in this, as they'll need to talk about things and get your advice and input, at least at first. But the exact role you play will depend in part on the age of your child – the older they are, the less they may want to involve you in knowing all the details of their abusive experience. Don't be surprised if, once your teenage child starts talking to a therapist, they become reluctant to divulge much information. Your role isn't to duplicate the work of a therapist or counsellor, but to be there for your child as and when they need it. You're their most intimate 'support group'. Your importance and uniqueness doesn't stem from *what you do*, but from *who you are*. So don't imagine for a moment that any therapist could take your place, and don't try to take theirs.

Lastly, don't imagine you have to go it alone any more than your child does. Abuse isn't one of those things a parent is expected to take in their stride. If you're not having trouble coming to terms with it, you're kidding yourself. So make sure you find someone – perhaps even another professional – to talk to about *your* feelings and *your child's* experience. If they're not a professional, try to ensure they're not too much out of their depth in talking to you and, above all, that you can rely on them to take whatever you say in the strictest confidence. Your child will be paranoid enough about people knowing – they don't need your friends inadvertently blabbing about town.

 **Top Tip:** *If your child has been sexually abused, involve Social Services – the abuse needs to be stopped – and find someone for both you and your child to talk it through with in confidence.*

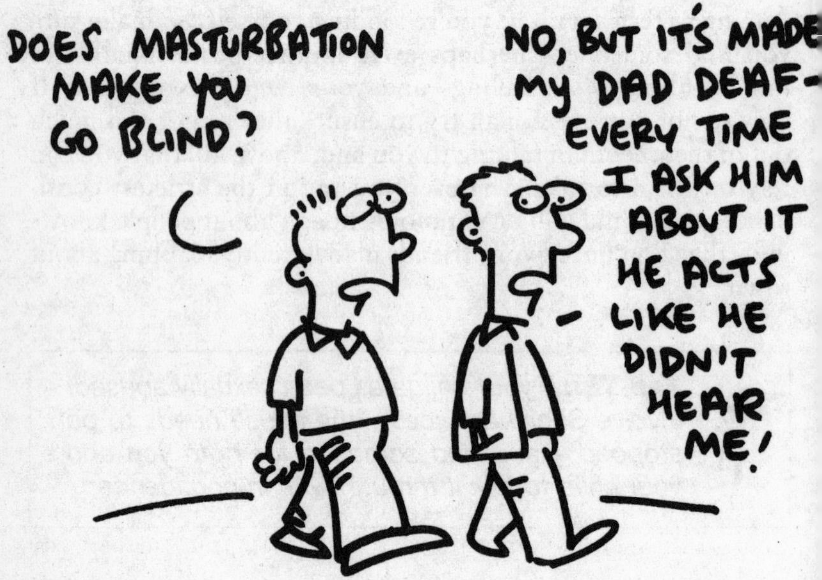
DOES MASTURBATION MAKE YOU GO BLIND?
NO, BUT IT'S MADE MY DAD DEAF- EVERY TIME I ASK HIM ABOUT IT HE ACTS LIKE HE DIDN'T HEAR ME!

# Mmmmmm . . .

## How to Broach the Issue
## of Masturbation

For some reason, masturbation is one of those things that rarely gets discussed in polite society, though it's the subject of volumes of toilet-wall poetry. It's also something that rarely forms an integral part of most parents' 'natural curriculum' when it comes to talking to their child about sex. In fact, it's right up there at the top of the list of the ten most embarrassing subjects ever to mention to your child.

It's strange, really. After all, survey after survey shows that masturbation is immensely common. Approximately 95 per cent of all men have masturbated at some point in their life, and the other five per cent were probably lying when they filled in the form! Nor is it just a male endeavour – over 60 per cent of women masturbate at one time or another. People can start masturbating as young as ten or eleven, sometimes even younger before they've even reached the age of puberty and developed sexually. And there's no upper age limit – you can masturbate until the day you die, though it's never been officially listed as a cause of death!

Single people, married people, divorced people, widowed people, gay people, straight people, white people, black people, old people, young people, parents, children: there probably isn't a socio-economic group on earth amongst whom masturbation is a non-event. But at the same time, there probably isn't a socio-economic group on earth prepared to own up and admit, 'Yep, we masturbate.' In other words, most of us do it – or have done it – but hardly any of us are willing to talk about it. The irony, of course, is that whilst none of us really *talk* about it, men in particular will happily *joke* about it, as long as they can do so without having to reveal the fact that they're speaking from personal experience!

As a result, adults – not to mention children – can end up believing that it's some kind of terrible and wicked perversion, and they're the only person in the whole wide world who does it, or ever has done it. They feel guilty, sure that everyone else on the planet would recoil in utter revulsion if only they knew the 'awful truth'. And if this is true of adults, it's *especially* true of children, who are acutely aware of every tiny difference between them and their friends when it comes to bodies and behaviour.

 **Top Tip:** *Even though research suggests that over 75 per cent of people masturbate, your child is likely to think they're the **only** one ever to have seriously thought about it.*

## Time to Start Learning Braille?

Masturbation is solo sex: stimulating your own penis or clitoris, usually until you reach a climax. Woody Allen once called it 'sex with someone you love'. But there are a lot of old wives' tales told about it, and your child is bound to come across some of them before long.

The most common masturbation myth is that it will make you go blind. The most bizarre one is that it will cause hair to grow on the palms of your hands. (If you see a blind werewolf stalking the streets . . .) Some people worry that masturbation makes you spotty, sterile or insane. Others consider it a source of disease or infection. The Victorians even believed that men could die as a result of what they discreetly termed 'solitary vices'. But the truth is, there's absolutely no evidence that masturbation is physically damaging. It's just one of the many misunderstandings your child may have picked up.

But some of these misunderstandings can be big causes of concern for children, especially once they enter the wonderful world of adolescence. So it's worth you taking the time to set some of your child's fears at rest and clear up their misapprehensions. By talking to them frankly and honestly, you'll be able to dispel some worrisome myths before they take root. The trouble is, this will inevitably mean *you* taking the initiative. Don't wait for it to crop up naturally in the conversation – it won't! You'll have to raise the issue 'out of the blue'.

It's very important at this point not to overdo it. It's the kind of thing you only want to talk about once, because it will actually be far more embarrassing for *them* than it is for *you*.

Try not to make it personal; instead, treat it as dispassionately and objectively as you can. Your child really doesn't need to know if you were a 'past master' at it yourself – nor will they want to! And the last thing you want to do is push your child into the kind of situation where they'll have to admit that they *do* (or *don't*) masturbate. Your goal isn't to tutor them for an MA in Masturbation. It's simply to dispel any fears they may have and give them a chance to clear up one or two misconceptions.

If all this seems just too much for you – or *them* – you may need to rely instead on a more indirect approach. Your local bookshop is bound to stock one or two good books about sex aimed at children or teenagers, and one of these is sure to cover the issue of masturbation. A few years ago I even wrote one myself, called *Sex Matters*, with a whole chapter devoted to this rather delicate subject. Just tell them that although you know it's a really embarrassing subject to discuss, you think it's such an important one for them to know about that you've bought a book for them to read on their own.

After all, the aim is *education*, not ritual humiliation. You don't want to come across like the Spanish Inquisition. You just want to lay some of your child's fears to rest and reassure them that they're not abnormal simply because they do – or don't – masturbate.

 **Top Tip:** As embarrassing as it seems, you'll need to raise the issue of masturbation yourself . . . either directly or by giving your child a book.

## Myth World

In other words, try to avoid turning a reassuring little chat into an hour-long seminar. If it's not too embarrassing for all concerned, you may be able to help bust a few of the myths. Apart from going blind and gradually turning into a human hairball, the top five masturbatory misconceptions your child is likely to encounter are:

- 'Wet dreams': Masturbation is different from a 'wet dream' (or 'nocturnal emission', as they're technically known) as it requires 'hands on' action. It also requires you to be conscious! 'Wet dreams' occur during sleep and are entirely out of a person's control. What's more, despite their name, you don't need to be dreaming about sex (or anything else) to get a 'wet dream'. In men, they're the result of an involuntary erection, when sperm seeps out of the penis. The female equivalent – a 'nocturnal orgasm' – involves fluid seeping from the vagina. Masturbation, by contrast, requires concentrated action, not to mention privacy, soundproofing and a spare five minutes!

- Blood pressure: As part of the arousal process in both men and women, blood flows to the genital area. If this state of arousal continues for some time, the accumulation of blood *can* cause a certain amount of genital discomfort. Orgasm is a way to relieve this discomfort, but it's by no means the *only* way – in fact, left to its own devices, with no more sexual stimulus, the body will return to the state it was in before arousal. Unejaculated sperm, for example, doesn't

129

*need* to 'escape', though it may do so in a 'wet dream'. It can just be reabsorbed by the body. In other words, there's no biological reason why someone *has* to masturbate or have sex. In the annals of recorded medical history, no one ever died as a result of non-masturbation!

- **Growth factor**: Boys, in particular, are apt to wonder whether masturbation can aid or accelerate the growth and development of their sexual organs. The simple answer is no. Though sex hormones are released in times of arousal, such as masturbation, these have no effect on physical development. Breasts and testicles, penis and pelvis will develop at their own rate, no matter how often a person masturbates.

- **Spent fuel**: Until the last century, doctors imagined we were born with a limited stock of sexual fluids (such as sperm) inside our bodies. As a result, we were advised not to squander them. Today, that theory is as dead as the doctors who devised it. The truth is that sperm, semen, eggs and vaginal fluid are all produced continuously in the body from puberty onwards. And except for eggs, which stop being made after menopause, production generally goes on for life. In other words, you can't 'use up' your sexuality, either by having 'too much' sex or by masturbating.

- **Future problems**: Some boys wonder if too much masturbation when they're young will lead to sexual 'performance' problems later on – will they reach orgasm too soon (the dreaded 'premature ejaculation'), or take too long? In fact, whilst masturbation can certainly be 'all over in a couple of minutes', this is no indication of how long sex will take with a partner. A number of factors govern the length of time it takes for a man to ejaculate with a partner, including hormones, menstrual cycle, lubrication, the amount of foreplay before penetration and the level of arousal of both partners. For a woman, too, masturbation doesn't automatically lead to problems achieving an orgasm, which tends to depend on how, and how much, her clitoris is stimulated during sex, regardless of whether or not she has a history of masturbation.

 **Top Tip:** *As a parent, you may be able to dispel some of the myths your child will probably have learnt about masturbation.*

### 'Forgive Me, Father, For I'm About to Sin . . .'

Of course, something isn't automatically *right* simply because it won't lead to later medical problems. To put it another way, just because your child won't need to get a new pair of prescription specs or start wearing gloves in public doesn't mean they should necessarily lock themselves in their bedroom with an industrial-size box of Kleenex and go all out for a new world record! Masturbation isn't a *medical* problem, but there are three important *moral* and *emotional* issues they'll need to consider.

1. **Guilt.** Like it or not, masturbation is a guilt-inducing activity, and society amplifies that guilt via the messages it

131

sends children about its rights and (more frequently) wrongs. For a long time, society strongly condemned masturbation as a 'mortal sin'. Today, we tend to avoid mentioning it if we possibly can. But this 'conspiracy of silence', added to the way we use terms like 'wanker' to insult people, actually reinforces the guilt most young people feel about masturbating.

2. **Obsession.** Some teenagers – especially boys – suspect that their behaviour borders on obsession. They're worried that their daily habit is becoming a dangerous addiction. But the truth is, whilst masturbation is clearly habit-forming – any urge so easy to satisfy can be habit-forming – it's very rare for it to be a real addiction. Addictions enslave or control you and tend to be accompanied by physical or emotional withdrawal symptoms. Of course, knowing that your 'nasty habit' just misses out on being a technical addiction isn't much comfort – after all, you've still got the habit. If you're trying to kick it, the traditional regimen of cold showers isn't the answer – it'll only give you hypothermia! The only thing that works is *distraction*: something else to occupy mind and body. Sexual energy is transferable: if it's not used for masturbation, it can be used for anything from marathon-running to marmalade-making!

3. **Dissatisfaction.** Sex is about communication. Ideally, it's about making yourself one with someone you love and trust. It's about the person you have sex with, not the sex itself. By contrast, masturbation is sex with yourself – no relationship, communication or intimacy. Ultimately, it's not 'the real thing'. It's a double act with only one player. That's why, more often than not, the frantic desires that lead to a

climax rapidly vanish afterwards. Instead of a sense of pleasant satisfaction, you're just aware of being alone. Guilt and glee turn to loneliness and boredom. It can become dangerous if this sense of dissatisfaction prompts your child to look for bigger thrills – and more satisfaction – in full-blown sex. It's not that there's anything wrong with sex. It's just that being bored with masturbation isn't a good reason for having it.

 **Top Tip:** *Just because masturbation won't kill you, that doesn't make it* right *– your child still needs to negotiate the moral and emotional maze.*

## Let Your Fingers Do the Walking . . .

There's one last aspect of masturbation to bear in mind: the mental side. Masturbation usually requires an element of sexual fantasy. It's rare for physical sensations alone to bring a person to climax, which is generally the goal of masturbation. And it's even more rare for a person to find sufficient erotic stimulation from the train timetable or the *Yellow Pages*. Whilst most people who masturbate rely on mental pictures from their memories and imaginations, some – especially men – need more visual or verbal stimulation. Often this means pornography.

Though some people argue that pornography is 'just a bit of fun', it actually cheapens both women and men. Of course, not all nude pictures or sex scenes in films and books are pornographic. As we saw earlier, many great works of art feature full-frontal nudity, whilst many classic works of literature aren't shy when it comes to sex. Even the Bible contains enough bonking to make you blush! The basic difference between nudity or sexual explicitness and pornography is that pornography is really only concerned with sex. It's not interested in the people having sex or the story in which they have it. In art and literature, sex plays a part; in pornography, it's all there is. Pornographic stories, films and photo shoots aren't interested in character, context, compassion or conversation. They're not out to win any Pulitzer Prizes – their sole purpose is to turn you on!

Pornography devalues people by turning them into sex objects rather than human beings. When a man stands with his tongue hanging out, gawping at a full colour centre-spread of a nude 'glamour' model, whatever it is he finds impressive, you can pretty much guarantee it isn't her personality! Pornography works by stimulating people's sexual desires, through either the written word or pictures. Women tend to be turned on more by atmosphere and imagination, which is more easily evoked by a piece of text than by photos. Men, on the other hand, tend to react more to blatant visual stimulation – the more blatant, the better.

The danger in all this is that it encourages us to think of other people as sexual objects – only there to help us reach orgasm – rather than as full human beings. Pornography makes sex into an item for sale, encouraging us to think of ourselves as sexual *consumers* rather than *contributors*. What becomes important to us isn't the other person's needs and desires, but simply having our own desires met – getting what *we* want.

Fantasy, of course, isn't just inevitable; it can even be healthy. We all fantasise, and our sex lives aren't exempt from this process. From Mills & Boon to Milton and Byron, the whole of world literature relies on our ability to put ourselves in someone else's shoes and live a different life for a few hours. The problem comes when our fantasies stop us enjoying the reality of what we've got and who we are. Even when it comes to having sex with a partner we love and find attractive, we can still find ourselves hankering after something – or some*one* – else.

In other words, whilst the physical sensations involved may be similar, masturbation and great sex are really opposites. Masturbation is a solo project, done for your own personal gratification; sex is a joint venture, in which the aim is to give pleasure to your partner. Masturbation is self-centred; sex is partner-centred. Masturbation may be good for the heart in purely cardiovascular terms, but it's a washout when it comes to good, old-fashioned love.

 **Top Tip:** *Masturbation encourages your child to see sex in terms of what their partner can do for them, not what they can do for their partner.*

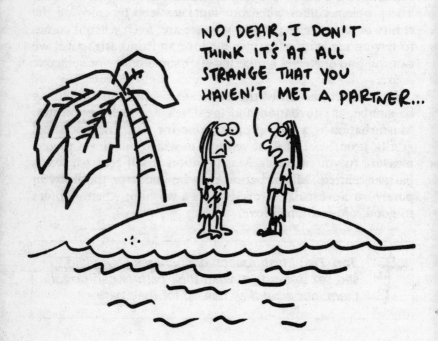

# Young, Free and Single

## What If Your Child Has
## No Boyfriend/Girlfriend?

What if your child hasn't got a boyfriend or girlfriend? Is this a cause for worry? Are they a freak? The simple answer to this question is no.

Women's and men's magazines are crammed full of articles on how to get your man or woman; how to make yourself irresistible; how to make yourself huggable; what to do with your partner once you've got them; how to satisfy them in bed; and what they most want sexually. The implicit assumption, at least as far as your child can see, is that the point of existence is to get (and perhaps even keep) a partner. Not having a boyfriend or girlfriend is more than just bad for their image – to a teenager it can seem like the unforgivable sin.

If your child has hit serious double figures and hasn't made it with the boy or girl of their choice, they may start to feel inferior. After all, 'real men' have no trouble attracting women, and 'attractive women' have no trouble getting a man. At least, that's what adverts and teen programmes seem to suggest. To your child, having a boyfriend or girlfriend can seem like the 'proof' that they're attractive or successful. It's a kind of status symbol, as if not having a partner proves you're a geek. You must be weak, or ugly, or both.

Faced with such pressures, your child may be tempted to 'get off with' the first available person of the right gender who doesn't look like *The Swamp Thing*. After all, they don't want to be a failure, and having a boyfriend or girlfriend – any boyfriend or girlfriend – seems to be an instant passport to success.

But is it really true that we need to be in a relationship with someone to be whole? Well, no! But whilst you know that, perhaps even from personal experience, your child may need a little more convincing. So, long before it becomes an issue for them – and they begin to suspect that you're only telling them about the satisfactions of the single life as a kind of consolation prize, because they can't get a boyfriend or girlfriend – it's important for you to take the time to look at some of the strange myths surrounding sex, snogging and singleness.

 **Top Tip:** *You know that having a boyfriend or girlfriend isn't the be-all-and-end-all of life, but your child may need some convincing.*

## 'Who's Gonna Love You When You're Old and Fat and Ugly?'

**Myth No. 1:** 'Having a partner proves I'm attractive.'

It's estimated, as we saw before, that around 80 per cent of teenagers don't like the way they look. Their nose is too big, their teeth are crooked, their ears stick out, their hair is the wrong colour, they're too fat, or their bum's the wrong shape, or their boobs are too big, or too small, or their stomach sticks out, or their legs are too fat, or too short, or too skinny, or their beard won't grow, or stop growing, or . . . well, you get the idea.

But who are they comparing themselves with? The truth is, not many of us are built like supermodels. Nor is there any reason why we should be. As Anita Roddick once pointed out, there are just eight supermodels in the world, and almost three billion other women. But because television and magazines are filled to bursting with beautiful, perfectly formed, size 10 women and muscle-bound, bronzed, handsome men, we tend to fall into the trap of thinking that this is the norm – the way we *should* be. Teenagers, and even pre-teens, aren't immune from these images or the feelings that go with them. 'If only I had a boyfriend or girlfriend,' they tell themselves, 'then I'd know I was attractive. And if I were attractive, I'd be happy.' But it's important to recognise three things:

1. *Supermodels don't really look like their photographs*. Without the two-hour make-up sessions, expert lighting, expensive clothes, flamboyant hairstylists, exotic locations, personal trainers and professional photographers – not to mention the 267 lousy shots needed just to get *one* printable one (which is often touched up afterwards, anyway, to remove any 'blemishes') – even supermodels look kind of . . . well . . . *ordinary*. Those who work in the fashion

industry know they're selling a fantasy, but half the time the rest of us believe it to be real.

2. *People we think of as stunningly attractive are rarely happy with their looks.* We might think film and pop stars are attractive, but they don't necessarily agree. In fact, some of them end up spending a fortune trying to improve their looks through diet, fashion and even surgery, fuelling tabloid debates as to how much of them is now made of plastic.

3. *Being attractive doesn't guarantee happiness.* Even looking like a supermodel doesn't guarantee you'll be any happier, or have more success in relationships, than the rest of us. Diana, Princess of Wales, was considered beautiful the world over, but her marriage still failed and some authors continue to make money trading on her sad life story. The lives of some film stars are just as tragic: in the 1950s, Elizabeth Taylor was one of the most beautiful women in the world, yet she's been married more times than most of us can count. And Marilyn Monroe, one of the most attractive women who ever lived, with a string of boyfriends that included US President John Kennedy, died lonely and scared, divorced from her third husband, having taken her own life by an overdose of sleeping tablets. At thirty-six, she just couldn't face living any more.

So the idea that having a partner means we're 'attractive', and being 'attractive' brings happiness, is plain wrong. The truth is, being 'attractive' isn't just about what we look like. It's about the whole package of *who we are* – our thoughts, interests, attitudes . . . in fact, everything that makes us *us*! Besides, even good looks are a matter of personal speculation rather than objective fact. Beauty, as they say, is in the eye of the beholder.

---

 **Top Tip:** *Having a boyfriend or girlfriend doesn't prove that your child is 'attractive', and being attractive won't guarantee their happiness.*

---

## 'The Man Who Has Everything'

**Myth No. 2:** 'Having a partner proves I'm successful.'

We all know how to recognise successful people. Their flash cars, Rolex watches and designer clothes are status symbols, announcing their success. But sometimes this kind of person even extends this idea to their relationships, picking partners who'll make them look good – like the power-dressed corporate executive who parades her toyboy in front of her friends or colleagues, or the middle-aged company boss with an expensively almost-dressed young blonde on his arm, less than half his age. 'Look at me,' they seem to be saying. 'I've got it all – a Porsche, a penthouse *and* a beautiful partner.'

Though they don't necessarily want the same status symbols, it's easy for your child to get trapped into this way of thinking: 'If only I had someone to go out with, then I'd be a success. I'd be worth something.' When you think about it, of course, this is a pretty silly idea. 'Success' doesn't lie in any of these things, and certainly doesn't guarantee happiness.

Alfred Nobel, the wealthy nineteenth-century inventor of

dynamite, detonators, smokeless gunpowder and gelignite was by anyone's standards a highly successful man – anyone's standards but his own, that is. Having devised his explosives for use in mining and road-building, Nobel had long been troubled by their lucrative military application. But he got the shock of his life one morning in 1888 when he found himself reading his own obituary in the newspaper. A careless journalist had unwittingly got him mixed up with his recently deceased brother, so Nobel had the rare chance to see how the rest of the world viewed him: a multi-millionaire merchant of death who had amassed a vast fortune from the weapons trade. Seeing the fruits of his 'success' summed up gave Nobel just the impetus he needed to ensure he'd be better remembered when his obituary was written for real. He set about changing his will so that, when he died, the bulk of his fortune went to fund the prizes that bear his name in physics, chemistry, medicine, literature and, of course, peace.

In other words, 'success', like beauty, is in the eye of the beholder. To many people, Nobel's wealth and achievements were symbols of undoubted success, but to him they were hollow reminders of how empty his life really was. In the same way, just having a partner isn't a good indicator of any 'success' worth having. Some of the world's most 'successful' people have also been some of the unhappiest. Elvis Presley was rich beyond his wildest dreams, world famous and married to a beautiful woman. But he, too, died of a drug overdose, bloated and in despair, at the age of just forty-two.

**Top Tip:** *Having a partner won't make your child a 'success' and can't guarantee their happiness.*

## 'I Can't Get No Satisfaction'

**Myth No. 3:** 'Having a partner will make me fulfilled.'

Being in a stable, loving relationship is undoubtedly a very fulfilling experience, but that doesn't mean you can only be fulfilled by going out with someone. Nor does it mean that just going out with someone – or even having a stable, loving relationship with them – will automatically be enough to fulfil you. Most of us find fulfilment through a combination of different things: our jobs, hobbies, achievements, interests, friends, family, faith.

Mother Teresa spent her life helping poor people in the slums of Calcutta. By anyone's standards she was an extremely successful, fulfilled woman. It wouldn't be an exaggeration, in fact, to call her a saint. Yet she never had a partner (it's against the rules for a nun!). Instead, she found fulfilment as a consequence of her decision *not* to have a partner. She'd never have achieved half the things she did in her life if she'd always had to get home by five o'clock in order to give Mr Mother Teresa his tea. So the idea that, if you're not in a relationship or going out with someone – *any*one – you're somehow going to end up being unfulfilled or unhappy just isn't true.

The truth is there are many thousands of people who are quite happy to be 'young, free and single'. Or even old, free

143

and single, come to that. And there are thousands more who regret having pinned their hopes of fulfilment on a relationship. Trevor Chambers, a 6 ft 3 in tall Australian with a long dark beard that would put even Chewbacca to shame, once gave passing shoppers a fright in Melbourne's central shopping centre by dressing up in a bridal veil with a tacky tiara of plastic pink flowers and wandering from one end of the mall to the other carrying a placard that read, 'Sex is not a cure for emptiness'. Even more surprising than the sight of a walking carpet in wedding gear was the reaction he got – man after man, woman after woman, came up to him and said, 'You're so right. I thought my partner would give me everything I needed, but they don't.'

The important thing to realise about these shoppers is that their *real* problem wasn't their partner but their unrealistic expectations. They'd gone into marriage expecting it to wave a magic wand, to make all their problems and loneliness disappear. But the reality is that periods of loneliness and feelings of isolation are a natural part of life. They can occur in the best of marriages as well as amongst single people. In fact, it's possible to be in an ideal marriage and *still* be unfulfilled, because fulfilment is never found in just one thing. Life is more complex than that, and true fulfilment is only ever found in a mixture of different things. If your child is under the impression that just finding a boyfriend or girlfriend is going to make them fulfilled overnight (sex or no sex), they're in for a very big shock.

---

 **Top Tip:** *Having a boyfriend or girlfriend won't suddenly make your child fulfilled – real fulfilment is only found in a combination of factors.*

---

## Fit Bodies, Fat Minds

So if your child isn't in a relationship – or better still, before they're old enough to consider a serious relationship – try to encourage them not to worry about being single and not to get too intense about it all. You don't want it to be allowed to take over their life.

They'd be better off using their time to learn new skills and to develop a wide range of interests. The way for them to broaden their appeal to others isn't by desperately trying to wish a boyfriend or girlfriend into existence – it's by becoming a more interesting and more fulfilled person. After all, their most powerful sexual organ is the one between their *ears*, not their *legs*. The friend at school who has no problems finding boyfriends or girlfriends, and who spends their time groping and bonking their way to popularity with the opposite sex (and often unpopularity with their own), can easily end up divorced and dissatisfied by the time they're thirty. By contrast, those who spend more time developing their interests are more likely to turn thirty with a sense of achievement and fulfilment.

In the long run, interesting people are more attractive than physically beautiful ones, especially when middle age sets in and, whoever you are, your assets head south and you begin to sag. If your child has learnt to develop genuine friendships with their own and the opposite sex, they'll find that they're able to be more relaxed and natural in their company, more skilled in the art of conversation, more rewarded by a wide circle of friends, more fulfilled as a person and, ironically, better equipped to form a lasting sexual relationship in the years to come. Above all, your child needs to avoid pinning their sense of self-worth on their attraction to the opposite gender and their success in getting a boyfriend or girlfriend. Even if they're successful, they'll only be disappointed.

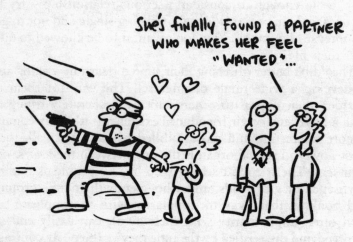

Sue's finally found a partner who makes her feel "wanted"...

**Top Tip:** If your child isn't in a relationship, try to help them see this as an opportunity to develop as a person, not as a sign of failure.

# A New Start

## How to Help Your Child
## Pick Up and Start Again

Life isn't like the cartoons. When Tom or Jerry hits a brick wall at sixty miles per hour, they go flat, fall backwards, then spring back to their original shape again a second later as if nothing had happened and just carry on, none the worse for wear. Unfortunately, it doesn't happen that way in real life.

If your child has just broken up with someone, or got far more intimately involved with them sexually than they'd intended, they're likely to be devastated. The pain of rejection, the chill of loneliness or the feelings of remorse and regret can have a very deep impact. They can feel ugly, used, unloved, unmotivated, unappreciated, unattractive and unlikely ever to find happiness ever again. And though it may seem like a temporary blip to you, it will probably seem like the end of the world to them. It's not something they can just calmly 'take in their stride' and get over in a day or two.

The chances are, you remember what it's like to feel this way from when it happened to you in your own teens, or perhaps more recently. The emotions don't change – though teenagers have far less life experience to fall back on than adults when it comes to knowing how to deal with these feelings.

This gives you a massive advantage ... an advantage you can pass on to your child. On the one hand, you want to support your child, letting them know that you care for them and that it really *isn't* the end of the world, however bad it might seem right now. On the other hand, you don't want to crowd them or cut short the grieving process they'll inevitably be going through. You want to give them advice, but you also want to give them time and space.

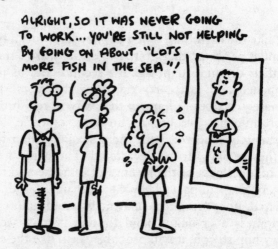

It's hard to watch the child you love feeling pain, but the truth is that the most valuable thing you can do for them in the first instance is just be there. Try not to fall into the trap of feeling you need to solve their problems for them – or even *with* them – and don't feel that you've got to keep talking just to fill in the silence. The truth is, we learn many of life's most valuable lessons through our struggles. If your teenager doesn't want to talk, don't force them to. Don't pry. If they want to be alone, make a discreet exit. If they want to cry, offer them your shoulder to cry on. Your presence alone is enough to help to reassure them that you love them, you haven't rejected them, and you're there to give them whatever support they need.

When the famous classical composer Robert Schumann died, his friend Johannes Brahms, another brilliant composer, visited Schumann's widow. But on arriving at the house, he just went straight to the piano, sat down, played a piece of music and left, without uttering a single word. It was the best way he knew to honour his friend and tell Mrs Schumann how he felt about her husband's death. He couldn't find any words to express his grief, but, of course, no words were really needed. The point was quite powerfully made without them. His presence was worth a thousand words. In the same way, you don't have to say much, and your child may not want to talk. But if they know you still love them unconditionally, it will help them to get things into perspective – even though the way they respond to you may not always show it.

The last thing they need from you at that moment is a lecture series. If you offer advice, make sure they're both willing and able to hear it. Otherwise, bite your lip. This is no time for saying 'I told you so', even if you did. And try to avoid telling them that you know how they feel because you went through 'exactly' the same experience when you were a teenager, even if it's true. They probably won't want to hear about it.

**Top Tip:** *If your child has broken up with some-one or made a mistake sexually, try to give them support and space. Be there, but don't crowd.*

## All's Well that Ends Well?

Ending relationships can be painful – and most of the common terms used to describe the break-up of a relationship reflect the various distorted ideas we've talked about throughout this book. People get 'dumped', 'dropped' or 'chucked' – as if what we were talking about was a discarded piece of rubbish, an object rather than a human being.

If your child has been dumped, therefore, they won't be feeling good about themselves. Your job is to help them see that *they're valuable for who they are, not who they go out with*. As much by being there as by saying anything, you need to reassure them that their value as a person doesn't stem from their 'fanciability', or their ability to form an early long-lasting relationship with someone. It stems from their utter uniqueness as a human being and the love their family and friends have for them.

Above all, however, they need to realise that, regardless of how bad or lonely they feel, if their relationship has broken up, they should resist the temptation to rush straight into another one. Relationships formed on the rebound often stem more from the need to find a replacement for the boyfriend or girlfriend they've lost, filling a gap in their life and taking away the loneliness, than from a real desire to be with the other person. That means your child will end up treating someone else like an object in just the way they themselves feel treated like one now. They'll probably end up stuck in a dead-end relationship they never really wanted in the first place, with a boyfriend or girlfriend they don't really respect – let alone love – simply because they needed to fill a temporary void in their life by embarking on a snogfest with the first available partner.

Ideally, your child needs to wait until they're less vulnerable before starting on something new. Spending time with friends, cooling off and mending their wounds – not to mention developing their interests and hobbies – is a much better way to regain their equilibrium. The next relationship should wait until they're sure they're entering into it because they like the person, not simply the fact of having a replacement boyfriend or girlfriend.

Above all, never tell your child that prospective partners are as plentiful as fish in the sea – when most of us go fishing, all we ever catch is an old boot! And don't compare the availability of boyfriends or girlfriends to the frequency of buses – the last thing you want your child to do is treat someone else like a No. 68, a means of getting from A to B!

---

 **Top Tip:** *If your child has broken up with someone, they should resist the temptation to leap straight into a relationship with someone else.*

---

### Dear John . . .

What if your child is the one ending the relationship?

One day they're madly in love, and the next day they wake up and the bubble has well and truly burst. Eros has packed

151

his bags and left. And now that the romantic fog that blinded them to each other's faults has lifted, they're struggling to understand what they ever saw in their boyfriend or girlfriend in the first place. How do they break up without giving their boyfriend or girlfriend a breakdown? Is there a way to split up and still retain a chance of being 'just good friends' afterwards?

Let's be honest: splitting is never an easy task. But having said that, there are one or two things your child can do to help ease the pain of the break-up for all concerned.

- **Be quick.** If your child is going out with someone and knows, in their heart of hearts, they're the wrong person, it's best not to keep them hanging on. Honesty may require a lot of courage, but it's far better than deceit. Beating about the bush, and putting off the inevitable moment, is easier in the short term, but it will result in all sorts of problems as time goes by, potentially leaving their 'ex' more hurt than ever.
- **Be clear.** If your child is breaking up with someone, especially if they still like them, it will help if they can explain _why_ they want to break up, letting the other person know just where they stand. Otherwise the 'dumpee' will have to furnish an explanation from their own imagination – and given the self-esteem levels of the average teenager, this is likely to be a recipe for future confusion and tortured self-doubt.
- **Be sensitive.** Being clear, firm and honest is one thing, but there are ways _to_ and ways _not to_ tell people things. It may be honest and accurate to tell someone straight-up that their breath smells worse than four-day-old camel dung slow-roasted over hickory coals, or that their new outfit makes

them look like Mr Bean, but there are more tactful and constructive ways of saying the same thing.

- **Be positive.** Most people only ever hear something about themselves if it's bad. It's like being summoned to the headteacher's office – you know if it happens that it isn't likely to be for anything good! So your child will be doing their former boyfriend or girlfriend a favour if they can explain not just what's *wrong* with them, but what's *right* with them as well – highlighting their good qualities, including what they found attractive about them in the first place. Your child will, however, need to avoid being patronising. Their former partner may be hurting, but they're not an object of pity.

- **Be open.** Above all, when breaking up with someone, it's best to give them plenty of room to speak. It will help if your child is willing to listen carefully to what their 'ex' has to say about themselves and the relationship. Apart from anything else, it's a sign of maturity for them to understand that, when relationships break up, the fault is never entirely one-sided. Even though the relationship is now over, there'll still be things your child can learn for the future.

> **Top Tip:** If your child is ending a relationship, it will help if they're quick, clear, sensitive, positive and open to the truth from another angle.

## 'Just Like Starting Over'

If your child has gone further than they intended sexually and done something they regret, they'll need in time to see that it's not the end of the world. They can begin again.

Of course, mistakes have consequences. And obviously, the more serious the mistake, the more serious the consequences may prove to be. But the important thing for any of us when we make mistakes is to learn from our experience, finding help if we need it and finding a way forward.

- If your child has had sex and thinks they may have become pregnant or contracted a disease, see your GP or another doctor. They're qualified to give the best possible help, and their advice will be confidential. If your child doesn't want you to go with them, or if you think they may be pregnant but they're unwilling to tell you about it, advise them to go to a Family Planning Clinic. That's what they're there for, after all.

- If they've had sex and feel used or disappointed, or even guilty, and they're reluctant to talk to you about it, it may help for them to talk to another adult they know and trust, or even a professional counsellor or organisation that specialises in counselling teenagers about sex. It's always good to talk things through with someone who's wiser and more experienced than you are, and who's not going to make any personal judgments based on what you say. In fact, confidentiality and non-judgmentalism are the key ingredients in finding a confidant.

Although they'll have to accept the emotional, social or physical consequences of their actions, you don't want your child to be trapped by their past or to think of themselves as soiled or second-hand goods. Nor do you want them to imagine that just because they've had sex once or twice, they might as well keep having it, even when they'd really rather not. It can be hard for young people to justify to themselves why they should say no another time if they've already said yes once. 'After all,' they may think, 'if I've lost my virginity, isn't the damage done? Isn't it too late?' But the truth is that it's *never* too late. Though virginity is something they can only give away once (and should therefore do only after having thought it through carefully), it's vital for your child to understand that they can learn and move on. They can begin again.

 **Top Tip:** *Your child needn't become a prisoner of their past – try to help them to learn from their mistakes . . . and move on.*

## The Eleventh Hour

Some people have sex because they feel that, having got to a certain point, they don't really have the right to back out. Perhaps they've been swept along by passion, much further than they'd have liked. They want to stop, but feel that wouldn't be fair to their partner. Perhaps they don't know how to call a halt. Or maybe, having consented to have sex with someone, they feel they've now got to go through with it. It may even have been their idea in the first place. But the truth is, it's never too late to make the decision not to have sex.

When the film *The Accused* came out in 1988, it stirred up a storm of controversy. It's the story of Sarah Tobias, a woman violently gang-raped in a bar, and her subsequent fight for justice against the men who raped her and the others who encouraged them. Many rape counselling services were unhappy with the film, since Sarah Tobias was far from the typical rape victim: drunk, stoned, provocatively dressed, sexually liberated, loud-mouthed and clearly looking for a good time, she even flirts with her attackers before her ordeal. Rape crisis centres were worried it would confuse the issue, but the film's defenders argued that it actually clarified the issue. Sarah Tobias, they suggested, had a *right* to flirt. She had a *right* to exhibit her sexuality in the way she dressed and danced. And she had a *right* to draw a line and refuse to have sex. Did she lead her attackers on? Perhaps. But that doesn't alter the fact that she had a legal and moral right to call a halt to the proceedings at *any* time. When her attackers and their supporters ignored this right, they turned a game of mutual flirting into a vicious rape.

In the same way, your child *always* has the right to draw a line and refuse to have sex. Whatever situation they're in, it's *never* too late for them to say no. All of us do silly things now and again, leading people on more than we should – perhaps we just don't think about the consequences of our actions, or perhaps we find the attention so flattering that we don't want it to stop. But as unwise as this kind of 'provocative' behaviour may be, it still doesn't alter the fact we have a legal and moral right to change our mind at *any* time – even halfway through, if things have got that far. So your child should *never* have to go through with something if they don't really want to. From the moment they say no, they've withdrawn their consent. And sex without consent, any way you cut it, is rape.

So what should your child do? How do they say no? The fairest and most effective way is for them to do exactly what an adult would do: push their partner away and shout (just to make absolutely sure they've heard), '*Stop! I don't want to do this!*' If necessary, they'll need to disentangle themselves and put their clothes back on. Gestures like this help reinforce the message that the 'fun' is genuinely over – the fat lady has now officially sung. The chances are, of course, that their partner won't be too pleased by this turn of events. In fact, they may need some convincing that your child is serious. But if they respect them, and don't want to find themselves in serious trouble, they *will* stop.

---

**Top Tip:** *Your child needs to understand that they have an absolute right to decide not to have sex at **any** time – even halfway through!*

---

## The Last Word

Your child's body belongs to *them*. No one else. Sometimes we feel pressured into doing things we'd rather not do, or things that, with hindsight, we'd rather not have done. And nowhere is this more true than when it comes to sex. It's easy for your child to be pushed into believing they're nobody unless they've 'done it', or that saying no to someone will make them unpopular. But your child's sexuality is a valuable gift, not a cheap toy for others to play with. That's why *they* need to be in control of what they do with it.

Your child needs to know that the responsibility for taking decisions about what they do with their body belongs to them. That's why it's important for them to have thought through their options early on, taking decisions about how far they're prepared to go *before* they get there, because waiting till it happens can be disastrous. If the moment is strong enough, they can end up going a lot further than they ideally want to before they really know what's going on. If they're relying on the telephone ringing, the CD finishing, their boyfriend or girlfriend suddenly changing their mind, parents returning home unexpectedly or the Pope appearing to them in a vision and warning them against the error they're about to make – anything to save them having to make the decision themselves – they're likely to be disappointed. And, in all probability, very sorry.

So as well as giving them all the biological, moral and emotional facts about sexual intercourse and development, the key message you need to instil in your child is this: it's their *right* to choose when, where, why, how and with whom they have sex. It's a choice they should make consciously and carefully, after full consideration of all the relevant facts and possible consequences. Sex is, after all, part of who they are. *They* should therefore be in control.

To help them retain this control, it's important to try to

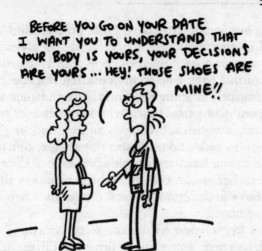

BEFORE YOU GO ON YOUR DATE I WANT YOU TO UNDERSTAND THAT YOUR BODY IS YOURS, YOUR DECISIONS ARE YOURS ... HEY! THOSE SHOES ARE MINE!!

establish an ongoing conversation with them from as early an age as possible. And you need to work hard at keeping this conversation going, especially through the difficult teenage years. This doesn't mean raising the subject of sex with predictable regularity every single chance you get. Nor does it mean collaring them the moment they get home from school, so they're afraid to walk through the door. If you did that with an adult, they'd draw the obvious conclusion that you're sexually obsessed and recommend you see a good psychiatrist. Don't think your child will be any different. Instead, it's important for you to strike a natural, healthy balance.

One of the advantages of this approach is that by the time they're a teenager – by the time bust-ups and sexual mistakes are on the cards – not only will you already have laid all the groundwork they'll need to help them make the necessary decisions, but you'll also have built up the kind of trusting relationship that will prove invaluable in giving them the sensitive support they'll need to cope with splits or mistakes.

Last month I took one of my children out for a meal in a local restaurant – nothing too fancy, just a chance for the two of us to spend some time together. It's something I try to do on a regular basis with each of my children, and it provides an opportunity to talk about all sorts of things, not merely sex. On this occasion, however, I took advantage of the situation to apologise to her in advance for all the mistakes I'm sure I'm going to make in the coming years, especially when it comes to the issue of boys.

'I wish I knew what to say on every occasion,' I told her, 'and how to react. But though I'm sure I'll get it wrong or embarrass you from time to time, I want you to understand that my real motivation is that I love you. If I seem to be hounding you or not trusting you, or if I say exactly the wrong thing at the wrong time, it's only because I'm concerned about you. I'm not trying to interfere. I'm just trying to help you make sense of it all. I know they're your decisions to make. I'd just like you to be able to make good ones, wise ones – ones you can live with, or even be happy with, ten or twenty years down the line.'

**Top Tip:** *Your child's body belongs to **them**, and **they** need to be the one making decisions about whether, when and with whom to have sex.*

# The 'Dirty Dozen':

## Twelve Awkward Questions Your Child Might Ask

## About Sex . . . and How to Handle Them

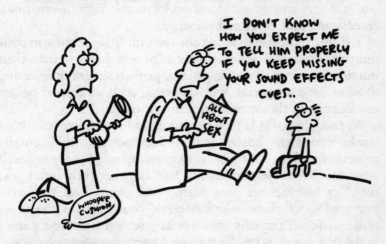

I DON'T KNOW HOW YOU EXPECT ME TO TELL HIM PROPERLY IF YOU KEEP MISSING YOUR SOUND EFFECTS CUES..

ALL ABOUT SEX

WHOOPEE CUSHION

### 1. Where do babies come from?

This, or something very like it, is probably the first question your child will ask you about sex. The chances are, they'll be three or four at the time. In other words, they're not a rocket scientist yet, so you don't have to give them a full colour, blow-by-blow description of the whole reproductive experience from hot'n'spicy foreplay to hospital forecourt. Just look on their first question as the start of a ten-year on/off conversation about sex, telling them enough to satisfy their curiosity but not too much for them to handle. Little and often is the best kind of approach. But whatever you do, don't save it all up for a big 'Sex Talk' when they're sixteen – by then it'll all be too late and too embarrassing. Above all, make your explanations as simple and straightforward as possible. You want your child to see sex and sexuality as a natural and valuable part of life, not a threatening and confusing minefield.

Tell them something along the lines of, 'Babies grow in their mummy's tummy.' When they ask how babies get *into* their mummy's tummy in the first place, explain that mummies and daddies have a 'special' way of loving each other, and babies are sometimes the wonderful result of that.

As tempting as it is to fob your child off with stories about storks, gooseberry bushes or birds and bees, all you'll actually achieve with this approach is to store up trouble for yourself later on. When they eventually find out the truth about sex, they'll wonder either how many 'little white lies' you were prepared to tell them in order to end your embarrassment, or how anyone as sexually ignorant as you ever became a parent in the first place! When Sam arrived home from school, he was furious. Summoning his parents to the living room, he announced in a loud voice, 'OK, let everyone in this house please stand advised that I, Samuel James Clarkson, have this day made a complete and utter fool of myself in sex education classes by repeating stories concerning storks told to me by certain parties residing herein!'

It's important to be truthful, but simplified. Anatomy isn't likely to be your child's strong suit, especially when they're four or five, and there's no reason why it should be. You want to tell them the truth, but there's no reason to tell them the *whole* truth *all at once*. When Corni and I taught our children to tell the time, for example, we didn't sit them down and explain in detail everything Einstein said about how time is relative to motion. (The main reason for this, of course, is that I don't have a clue myself!) Instead, we told them about the big hand and the little hand and all the numbers in between. The rest could wait. We slowly told them more and more as they got older and were able to take it in.

Truth may be stranger than fiction, and much more embarrassing to deal with, but in the long run it'll be a lot more useful to your child. For one thing, it'll give them a firm factual basis on which to build a proper understanding of sex. For another, it'll help protect them against some of the more persistent and pernicious myths surrounding sex by arming them with an informed, no-nonsense approach – after all, knowledge is power.

## 2. Do you really do *that* . . . and do *I* have to do it when I'm older?

When Sarah's young son asked what the two people on the television screen were doing, she replied that they were giving each other a 'special cuddle' – the kind that makes a baby.

'Oh,' he replied, 'I thought that happened when the man put his penis into the woman's vagina!' Like it or not, all children are now routinely exposed from quite a tender age not just to sexual images – on everything from billboards to broadcasts – but also to sexual information. When they finally grasp the full reality of what sex is, your child is more likely to be revolted by the prospect than to relish it, especially if they're still nine or ten. Most children move through a long phase of bonding with their own gender – boys think girls are weak, girls think boys are stupid. The idea of intimate contact with the opposite gender is about as appealing as munching on maggots.

This is a good time to help your child begin to understand about the emotional and moral aspects of sex, if you haven't already done so, passing on your values to them. It's also a good time to explain about the effects that hormones will have on their desires, as well as making sure they understand the concept of consent (including rape and sexual abuse). In particular, it's a good time to help them understand that sex and sexuality are basically a *good* thing.

If they seem especially afraid of or repulsed by the prospect of having sex, ask them as sensitively as you can if they've ever been touched by anyone in a way they don't feel comfortable with. Make sure they realise they can always talk to you if anyone – anyone *at all* – ever does touch them in a way they're uncomfortable with.

### 3. When are you too young to have sex?

Although a girl is physically ready for sex just before her first period, and a boy once he starts getting erections, the truth is that this is almost always much too young emotionally. Most children instinctively realise this, in spite of the fact that their hormones have started going haywire and confusing matters. Society as a whole recognises it, too, by setting the minimal age of consent at sixteen. (At the time of writing, the age of consent for gay males is eighteen.) Below this age, young people aren't judged to be emotionally mature enough to make their own responsible sexual choices. The fact remains, however, that 25 per cent of boys and 20 per cent of girls have sex under the age of sixteen. What's more, many of those over sixteen aren't really mature enough to make their own wise and responsible decisions.

So it's not enough just to tell your child that 'under sixteen' is too young to have sex. It's important to explain to them *why* there's an age of consent, helping them develop the kind of bigger picture they'll need if they're going to be ready and able to make good choices for themselves once they turn 'sweet sixteen'. They'll need to know the difference between a good choice and a bad choice, as well as how to resist the various pressures put on them to have sex before they really feel ready – before it's genuinely their *own* choice. Don't try to make their decisions for them, or present them with an easy answer. Instead, concentrate on giving them the emotional equipment and factual information necessary for their own choice to be a good one, and then make it clear that you trust them. Don't worry that this kind of briefing will push them into having sex early – all the evidence suggests that a good sex education (including the how-not-tos as well as the how-tos) actually pushes the age of first contact *up*, not down.

## 4. Does sex hurt?

If your child is still relatively young when they ask you this, they've probably come across a sex scene on TV and misunderstood what all the synchronised grunting and groaning is about. The simple answer is no. If they're a bit older, and you're already explaining all the ins and outs of sexual intercourse to them, it's time to answer this question more fully. Sex *can* hurt, but it usually only hurts in women and means one of three things:(a) she's having sex for the first time, and her hymen hasn't yet broken; (b) there's some inflammation around the vagina, a result of anything from stress to infection (it's worth seeing a doctor); or, (c) penetration is happening too early in the proceedings, before the vagina is sufficiently lubricated.

## 5. Is there anything wrong with me? Am I abnormal?

As the old saying goes, 'It's not what you've got that counts; it's what you do with it.' But for the majority of teenagers, struggling to come to terms with the changes in their bodies, size is *everything*. To be more accurate, being roughly the same size and shape as everyone else is everything. Nothing is worse for a teenager than being the first or last one amongst a group of friends to develop. If a girl is 'too big' or 'too small' up top, it can be crushingly embarrassing. If a boy's voice is the first or the last to break, or if his facial hair is quicker or slower to grow than everyone else's, he can feel like a freak. To the teenage mind, average is everything. Unsure of themselves and uncertain of being accepted by their peers, they rely on the safety of numbers.

As a parent, however, it's your job to help them come to accept who and what they are in themselves. In 1943, in the midst of the Second World War, US pastor Reinhold Niebuhr scribbled a short prayer on the back of an envelope in a small New England village church. Famous, thanks to its adoption by Alcoholics Anonymous, it reads: 'God give us grace to accept with serenity the things that cannot be changed, courage to change the things that should be changed, and the wisdom to distinguish the one from the other.' As a mum or dad, this is the kind of attitude you want your child to adopt when it comes to how they see themselves when they look in the mirror.

Their size, shape, sex, colour and weight bracket, for example, are all encoded in their genes, and short of radical surgery there's not much they can do about them. The more you can help your child see these things in a positive light, learning to accept and even treasure them, the happier they'll be in the long run. In fact, it's the very characteristics that make them different from everyone else that are so special. So by helping your child develop the wisdom to know what they should and shouldn't try to change about themselves, you'll be helping them become a unique, and uniquely valuable, individual.

## 6. How do I say no?

Knowing their own mind is vital for any teenager, but having the courage to stick to their decisions is every bit as crucial as knowing how to make them in the first place. As a mum or dad, you don't want your child being pressured into doing something sexually they don't want to do, so it's vital for you to help them say no if they don't want to have sex. In part, this comes down to explaining to them what their range of options is and what the possible consequences of choosing each option might be. It's important for you not just to explain the option *you* want them to take, but to educate them carefully and calmly about *all* the options. After all, they're constantly surrounded by sexual information, much of it one-sided and inadequate. If you don't tell them about the other options, the chances are they'll hear about them from someone else, only in a dangerously incomplete version.

As well as education, however, you'll need to help your child develop the self-confidence and self-esteem needed to stand up for what they believe in. It's not easy to say 'no' or 'not yet' to sex when so many others seem to be saying 'yes, yes, yes'. It takes a lot of courage and, nine times out of ten, it also takes a lot of moral support. Some of this support should come from their friends, but your child will also need to know that you're backing them all the way. Unconditional, no-strings-attached love is a key ingredient in giving them the sense of self-worth they'll need if their decision is going to be not just their own, but also a wise one.

## 7. How far should I go?

The simple answer is, only as far as they feel entirely comfortable going and, of course, always within the law. But unless you keep your child radio-tagged and under 24-hour surveillance, telling them how far to go isn't going to be much use. It has to be *their* decision, not *yours*, if they're to stand any chance at all of sticking to it in the heat of passion. They'll need to feel a sense of 'ownership' of it. That's why it's so important for you to make sure you pass on your values to your child as a framework for them to think through where they should stand on all the issues as carefully as possible beforehand. Only then will they be sure about how far they want to go and why. It's no good their trying to make up their minds on the spot. It'll be hard enough for them not to overstep their limits if they've carefully thought them all through themselves beforehand. If they *haven't* set any limits beforehand, they're likely to end up going much further than they really wanted to. Desire is a major motivator, and it's almost impossible to think straight in the heat of the moment.

Make sure your child understands some of the consequences of going to various different stages – kissing, cuddling, petting, heavy petting, penetrative sex – and explain about the emotional consequences, not just the mechanical ones. Then trust your child to make up their own mind, leaving the door open for them to talk again in the future if they choose to. If they know it's their decision, and they know why they made it – and you've done everything you can to help them develop a healthy self-confidence – they're likely to stick to it, even when every hormone in their body tells them not to.

No one said sticking to a decision was easy, of course. The problem is that we're often torn: part of us wants to say yes, another part wants to say no. It all comes down to long-term versus short-term desires. In the long term, we want everything to be absolutely perfect: the timing, the atmosphere, the partner, the passion, the whole shebang. We want to be able to look back and be really glad that we did what we did when we did it. But in the short term, even when the conditions and the partner are very far from perfect, we can still *really* want to have sex. Primed by our hormones and propelled by our desire, it's very confusing to feel two equal and opposite desires at one and the same time. To be strong or not to be strong: that is the question.

It's important to prepare your child for the full reality of this dilemma, or they can all too easily end up doing something they later regret. The truth is, they *can* stop – if they really want to. But the longer they put off making that tough decision, with their tongue surgically implanted in their boyfriend or girlfriend's mouth and their hands fumbling nervously with buttons and bra straps, the tougher it'll be to make the right decision. Swept along by a tide of passion, they'll find it almost impossible to make a clear, conscious, calculated choice. They'll also tend to ignore the whole issue of protection and 'safer sex'.

## 8. Can you get pregnant the first time?

According to all the statistics, the most dangerous category of driver in the UK isn't the befuddled senior citizen whose milk-bottle-bottom glasses haven't been cleaned in months, but young men within a year or two of having passed their test. The combination of too much confidence in their own abilities, too little experience of the stupid things that other drivers can do and an inadequate knowledge of the highway code too often proves to be lethal. In the same kind of way, young people's over-confidence that 'it could never happen to me', their ignorance of the risks and possible consequences of their actions, their failure to take proper precautions, their lack of experience in using contraceptives effectively and their relative emotional immaturity can sometimes combine to produce disastrous results.

Your child needs to know the truth about contraception and the risks of contracting a sexually transmitted disease (STD). For their own protection, they need to be informed and in control. So sit down quietly with them and explain all the various forms of contraception. It'll be embarrassing, of course – even more so for them than you. But it's vital for you to help your child understand the potential pleasures and pitfalls of sex. It can be wonderful, but it can sometimes also be lethal. And for 8,000 under-sixteens each year, it can be an unexpected introduction to instant motherhood. So make sure your son or daughter understands the risks of pregnancy or catching an STD the first time and *every* time. And make sure they know about the full contraceptive range, including what Woody Allen once called the ultimate 'oral contraceptive': the word 'no'.

## 9. How do I know I've picked the right person?

This is never an easy question to answer. Most of us, at heart, want the fairy tale. We want to find someone who makes our heart beat that little bit faster, who loves us for who we are with no strings attached, and with whom we'll spend the rest of our lives. We also, if we're honest, want them to be drop-dead gorgeous. But that's quite a demanding package, and it's not one we're guaranteed to find instantly, if at all. What's more, it's a package that changes as we grow older, because *we* change as we grow older. That's why the kind of partner we look for when we're fourteen is very different from the kind of partner we look for when we're forty. It's also why some couples break up: if you're not working to ensure that you're growing together over the years, you're bound to end up growing apart.

In other words, the key qualities your child needs to look for in a possible partner aren't lip-smacking lusciousness or spine-tingling sensuality, but love, support and 'reconcilable differences'. They don't need to look for someone exactly like them, nor do they need to branch out in the belief that 'opposites attract'. What really matters is that their boyfriend or girlfriend is someone who brings out the best in them, and with whom they really can be 'themselves'. Their differences should complement one another, and the things they have in common should help them to support and encourage one another.

The chances are, your child will have at least one or two relationships before they find the person they feel is Mr or Ms Right. This isn't necessarily a bad thing, and they don't need to go into every relationship thinking, 'This is the one!' In fact, having such high expectations can stop them from appreciating their boyfriend or girlfriend for who they are. Not every relationship has to last forever, and few relationships that begin in the teen years do last forever. But that makes it all the more important for your child to think very carefully about how far they want to go sexually with their present girlfriend or boyfriend. They can't have their cake and eat it. The more sexually experienced they become outside an exclusive lifelong relationship, the more difficult it will be for them to make sex with the man or woman of their dreams (when they finally find them) an intimate, private, personal and exclusive thing.

## 10. What if I never find a boyfriend or girlfriend?

Never is a very long time, and there's no way your child will fully understand the idea that they may not meet someone worth going out with until they're in their twenties or thirties. Turning sixteen or seventeen without having had a boyfriend or girlfriend feels like being left on the shelf as unwanted goods. Your child is likely to start imagining all sorts of things 'wrong' with them if they're progressing steadily through their teens and haven't yet played tonsil hockey with at least one boy or girl. As their mum or dad, it's your job to reassure them there's nothing wrong with them, and persuade them not to end up dating *anyone* just so they can say they've been out with *someone*.

Laurence Olivier, the world-famous actor, once admitted in an interview that he hadn't always chosen the film jobs he'd done for purely 'artistic reasons' – sometimes the money he'd been offered had been too tempting to turn down, even though the film was dire. With hindsight, he wondered about the wisdom of accepting these jobs, as the brilliant work he'd done in one or two of his films was in danger of being obscured by the sheer volume of bad acting he'd done. In the same way, it's good for your child to be discriminating about who they go out with, rather than dating the Grim Reaper just because they're free on Saturday night. It's better to spend time with a wider group of friends, developing your interests, than date someone you're not interested in just because there doesn't seem to be a better candidate.

## 11. How do I cope with rejection?

At some point in their life, your child is almost guaranteed to be unceremoniously 'dumped' by a boyfriend or girlfriend. It won't be pleasant, but it won't be the end of the world. It'll just *seem* like it at the time. Most couples break up because the things they have in common are no longer as obvious as the differences between them. As they get to know one another, the tingle-up-the-spine magnetic attraction they initially felt for each other begins to fade, and they get to see more clearly what they like and dislike about each other. When the likes are outweighed by the dislikes, and the magnetic attraction isn't strong enough to keep them together, they split. To you, it's obvious they just weren't right for each other, but to your child the only thing that's obvious is that someone they care about has seen what they're really like and rejected them.

In order to help your child recover, it's important to let them see how much *you* love them – though it won't seem like much of a consolation at the time – and to reassure them that it wasn't a fault in *them*, but a mismatch in the relationship, that caused the break-up. Whatever you do, *don't* tell them there are 'plenty more fish in the sea' – it'll sound patronising and simply convince them you just don't understand what's happened to them. Instead, give them the space to go through a process of bereavement for the 'dead' relationship. They'll need you to be there for them, but don't imagine you can 'kiss it better' as you used to do with a graze, or say something that will instantly make them feel better. The only advice you can really give them, if necessary, is *not* to start a new relationship when they're still on the 'rebound'.

## 12. I think I've made a mistake – what now?

We all make mistakes, and love is no exception. If your child does something sexually that, in the cold light of day, they wish they hadn't, you can play a vital part in helping them learn from their experience and move on. The first thing to realise is how privileged you are if they feel close enough to share this with you – and that it's absolutely vital for you *not* to repay their trust by leaping to judgments. They don't need you to tell them how stupid they've been – they already know that. What they need instead is unconditional love and acceptance. They need to know that whatever they've done, you still can't help loving them and you'll always be there to support them.

The next thing they need to know is that, however bad things are, it's not the end. Even though they may have to live with the full consequences of their actions – pregnancy, for example, or the knowledge that they've hurt somebody else very badly –

they can still begin again. They don't have to be a prisoner of their past. Above all, never let your child think of themselves as soiled or second-hand goods. The people who care about them will forgive them their mistakes. Instead, help them to learn from these mistakes, turn the page and move on. Encourage them to think through their options, take decisions about how far they want to go in the future, and begin again as if with a clean sheet.

# Further Information

## Organisations

### Parentalk
PO Box 23142
London SE1 OZT

Tel: 020 7450 9073
Fax: 020 7450 9060
e-mail: info@parentalk.co.uk
Website: www.parentalk.co.uk

*Provides a range of resources and services designed to inspire parents to enjoy parenthood.*

### Fathers Direct
Herald House
Lambs Passage
Bunhill Row
London EC1Y 8TQ

Tel: 020 7920 9491
Fax: 02 7374 2966
e-mail: enquiries@fathersdirect.com
Website: www.fathersdirect.com

*An information resource for fathers.*

### Gingerbread
7 Sovereign Close
Sovereign Court
London E1W 3HW

Advice Line (freephone): 0800 018 4318 (Mon–Fri, 9.00 a.m.–5.00 p.m.)
Tel: 020 7488 9300
Fax: 020 7488 9333
e-mail: office@gingerbread.org.uk
Website: www.gingerbread.org.uk

*Provides day-to-day support and practical help for lone parents.*

### Health Development Agency
Holborn Gate
330 High Holborn
London WC1V 7BA

Publications Line: 0870 121 4194
Tel: 020 7430 0850
Fax: 020 7061 3390
e-mail: communications@hda-online.org.uk
Website: www.hda-online.org.uk

*Produces a wide range of leaflets and other useful information for families on a wide variety of topics.*

**Home Start UK**
2 Salisbury Road
Leicester LE1 7QR

National Information Line
  (freephone): 08000 68 63 68
Tel: 0116 233 9955
Fax: 0116 233 0232
e-mail: info@home-start.org.uk
Website: www.home-start.org.uk

*Provides trained, parent volunteers
to help any parent with at least one
child under five, who is finding it
hard to cope.*

**Kidscape**
2 Grosvenor Gardens
London SW1W 0DH

Tel: 020 7730 3300
Fax: 020 7730 7081
e-mail: info@kidscape.org.uk
Website: www.kidscape.org.uk

*Works to prevent the abuse of
children through education programmes involving parents and teachers,
providing a range of resources. Also
runs a bullying helpline.*

**One Parent Families**
255 Kentish Town Road
London NW5 2LX

Helpline (freephone): 0800 018 5026
Tel: 020 7428 5400
Fax: 020 7482 4851
e-mail: info@oneparentfamilies.
  org.uk
Website: www.oneparentfamilies.
  org.uk

*Information service for lone parents.*

**National Drugs Helpline**
Frank
Freepost
PO Box 4000
Glasgow G3 8XX

Tel: 0800 776600
Website: www.talktofrank.com

*Free helpline offering confidential
advice. Can also send out free leaflets and answer any queries callers
might have.*

**National Family and Parenting Institute**
430 Highgate Studios
53–79 Highgate Road
London NW5 1TL

Tel: 020 7424 3460
Fax: 020 7485 3590
e-mail: info@nfpi.org
Website: www.nfpi.org

*An independent charity set up to
provide a strong national focus on
parenting and families in the 21st
century, they have a network of local
centres offering a range of services
for parents and children.*

**NSPCC**
Weston House
42 Curtain Road
London EC2A 3NH

Tel: 020 7825 2500
Helpline: 0800 800 500
Fax: 020 7825 2525
e-mail: help@nspcc.org.uk
Website: www.nspcc.org.uk

*Aims to prevent child abuse and neglect in all its forms and gives practical help to families with children at risk.*
*The NSPCC also produces leaflets with information and advice on positive parenting – call 020 7825 2500.*

**Parentline Plus**
520 Highgate Studios
53–76 Highgate Road
Kentish Town
London NW5 1TL

Helpline (freephone): 0808 800 2222
textphone (freephone): 0800 783 6783
(Mon–Fri, 9.00 a.m.–5.00 p.m.)
Fax: 020 7284 5501
e-mail: centraloffice@parentlineplus.org.uk
Website: www.parentlineplus.org.uk

*Provides freephone helpline called Parentline and courses for parents via the Parent Network Service. Parentline Plus also includes The National Stepfamily Association. For all information call the Parentline freephone number above.*

**Positive Parenting**
2A South Street
Gosport PO12 1ES

Tel: 023 9252 8787
Fax: 023 9250 1111
e-mail: info@parenting.org.uk
Website: www.parenting.org.uk

*Aims to prepare people for the role of parenting by helping parents, those about to become parents and also those who lead parenting groups.*

**Relate: National Marriage Guidance**
Herbert Gray College
Little Church Street
Rugby CV21 3AP

Tel: 01788 573 241
or lo-call 0845 456 1310
Fax: 01788 535 007
e-mail: enquiries@national.relate.org.uk
Website: www.relate.org.uk

In Northern Ireland:

76 Dublin Road
Belfast BT2 7HP

Tel: 02890 323 454

*Provides a confidential counselling service for relationship problems of any kind. Local branches are listed in the phone book.*

**The Trust for the Study of Adolescence**
23 New Road
Brighton BN1 1WZ

Tel: 01273 693 311
Fax: 01273 679 907
e-mail: info@tsa.uk.com
Website: www.tsa.uk.com

*Working to help improve the lives of young people and families and increase knowledge and understanding about adolescence and young adulthood.*

**Wired for Health**
Website: www.wiredforhealth.gov.uk

*Wired for Health is a series of websites managed by the Health Development Agency on behalf of the Department of Health and the Department for Education and Skills.*

# More About Paren**T**alk

Launched in 1999, in response to research, which revealed that 1 in 3 parents feel like failures, Parentalk is all about inspiring parents to make the most of their vitally important role.

A registered charity, we exist to provide relevant information and advice for mums and dads in a format that they feel most comfortable with, regardless of their background or family circumstances.

Our current activities include:

- **The Parentalk Parenting Principles Course**
  Already used by almost 25,000 mums and dads, this video-based resource brings together groups of parents to share their experiences, laugh together and learn from one another. Filmed at the studios of GMTV, endorsed by the National Confederation of Parent Teacher Associations and featuring Parentalk Founder Steve Chalke, the course is suitable for use by groups of parents in their own homes or by schools, PTAs, pre-schools and nurseries, health visitors, health centres, family centres, employers, churches and other community groups.

- **Parentalk Local Events**
  Looking at every age group from the toddler to the teenage years, and from how to succeed as a parent to how to succeed

as a grandparent, Parentalk evenings are a specially tailored, fun mixture of information, shared stories and advice for success as a mum, dad or grandparent. Operating across the country, the Parentalk team of speakers can also provide input on a range of more specialist subjects such as helping your child sleep or striking a healthy balance between work and family life.

- **Parentalk at Work Events**
  Parentalk offer lunchtime and half-day workshops for employers and employees, at their place of work, that look at getting the balance right between the responsibilities of work and those of a family. Parentalk also provides a life coaching service for employees, helping them to deal with the pressures they encounter at home in order to be happier, and perform better, at work.

  All Parentalk at Work initiatives are backed up by a comprehensive website: **www.parentalk.co.uk/atwork**

- **The Parentalk Guide Series**
  In addition to the 'How to Succeed' series, Parentalk offers a comprehensive series of titles that look at a wide variety of parenting issues. All of these books are easy-to-read, down-to-earth and full of practical information and advice.

- **The Parentalk Schools Pack**
  This resource, designed especially for year 9 pupils, builds on the success of the Parentalk Video Course, to provide material for eight lessons on subjects surrounding preparing for parenthood. The pack has been tailored to dovetail with

the PHSE and citizenship curriculum and is available for teachers to download from the Parentalk website.

- **www.parentalk.co.uk**
  www.parentalk.co.uk is a lively, upbeat site exclusively for parents, packed with fun ideas, practical advice and some great tips for making the most of being a mum or dad.

To find out more about any of these Parentalk initiatives or our plans for the future, or to receive our quarterly newsletter, contact a member of the team at the address below:

**Parentalk**
115 Southwark Bridge Road
London SE1 0AX
Tel: 020 7450 9073
Fax: 020 7450 9060
e-mail: info@parentalk.co.uk

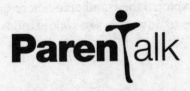

**Helping parents make the most of every stage
of their child's growing up.**

*(Registered Charity No: 1074790)*

## When Opposites Attract . . .

# Sex Matters

### Steve Chalke and Nick Page

- Why is sex such a big seller today?
- Is it all it's cracked up to be?
- What difference does love make?
- What happens when love and sex get separated?
- Is marriage the same as living together?
- Are there limits in sex?
- What do you look for in a partner?
- How do you control your sex drive?

*Sex Matters* explores these and many more questions while offering practical advice on sex and relationships to young people.

Published by Hodder & Stoughton
ISBN 0 340 65661 1